BABIES BORN EARLY

A GUIDE FOR PARENTS OF BABIES BORN BEFORE 32 WEEKS

DR WLODZIMIERZ M. WISNIEWSKI

Medical disclaimer

The information provided in this book is only for general educational purposes. The book is not meant to be used—nor should it be used—to diagnose or treat any medical condition. For diagnosis, treatment of any medical condition, and decisions regarding your health and that of your family members, you need to consult your physician. Furthermore, neither I nor the publisher can give you assurances or warranties that—at the time of purchase—information in the book was totally accurate and up to date.

Table of Contents

Thank you!

I dedicate this book to my parents and my wife, Mary. They always believe in me and support me in all difficult moments.

I want to thank all the families of my little patients whom I have had the privilege to meet over the past 30 years. I assure you that I continuously learn from each encounter. Thanks to you, I improve my social and medical skills every time. I always listen to my parents in the same way that I listen to my nurses. There were numerous instances when parents spotted something that neither I nor my nurses had seen, thereby contributing to better care for their baby. You always prove to me that more knowledgeable parents equal better outcomes for babies.

I also want to thank all my teachers, professors, and professional colleagues from Poland and the USA. I will only mention four names here, but I can assure you that there are at least 30 others deserving of mention. Thanks to Dr Wojczak, I began my career as a pediatrician 30 years ago in Poland. Dr Grzelak was a chief neonatologist in Kalisz Children's Hospital (Poland), where I began my training as a neonatologist. She and her team gave me initial training in this challenging specialty. Finally, thanks to professors J. Gadzinowski (Poznan Medical School, Poland) and D. Vidyasagar (University of Illinois at Chicago [UIC]), I had the opportunity to come to Chicago and study pediatrics and neonatology at the UIC. I was blessed with having excellent teachers in my life. They all influenced me not only as a doctor but as a human being. Now, I am trying to repay that by teaching and educating other young doctors and families of my patients.

Finally, I want to thank my editor Anne Abel Smith. Without her help this book would not have been possible.

CHAPTER 1

Introduction

Every year, approximately 380,000 babies in the USA and 15 million worldwide are born prematurely. Prematurity places a huge burden on each affected family because many babies need to stay in hospital for a long time after birth. Despite our best efforts as healthcare providers, we are unable to ensure the survival of all babies, or, if they survive, that all of them will have a healthy childhood and normal development.

These factors have a negative influence on affected families. Stressed-out parents are always anxious and fearful for the lives of their preemies. Over the past 20 years of my career as a neonatologist, I have seen parents sitting up all night at the bedside of their child in the neonatal intensive care unit (NICU) and reading on the internet about the various conditions affecting them. However, parents often told me that those resources were inadequate. Blog posts, or even articles published by reputable institutions, either lacked the breadth of knowledge or glossed over any unpleasant information. Also, because of a mandate on public institutions that medical information should be understandable and accessible to all people, articles are often written in language appropriate for 5th-graders.

In this book, I have decided to overcome those shortcomings. I will give you a lot of medical information regarding conditions in premature babies, their therapies, and their prognoses. The journey of a newborn baby in the NICU, from birth until discharge home, will be explained. However, that means I can't avoid using a little more "medical jargon" than you are probably used to seeing in books for parents. Still, I think the book will be easily readable and digestible for anybody with high school or college education. After reading the book, please send me your feedback by email (info@neopededu.com) or via my Facebook page (NeoPedEdu). That way, I will be able to improve my approach in any future editions. If you want to ask a question or have me clarify something you have read in the book, post that on my Facebook page too. I will do my best to answer it, but I will not be able to discuss anything related to your baby's condition because that could be construed as giving you medical advice, which is not my intention.

I am a firm believer that knowledge gives one power. For me, even scary information is better than uncertainty. While writing this book, I have been thinking of *you*—parents—who unexpectedly happen to have a premature baby who will require a long stay in a NICU. Knowing more about prematurity, you will feel empowered to participate in your conversations with the doctors in the unit. You are likely to encounter situations when you will have to choose between different diagnostic or treatment options. You will probably be asked to give consent for a treatment, procedure, or surgery. Existing knowledge about conditions affecting premature babies will allow you to ask the right questions and decide on the right path for your baby.

Who shouldn't read my book?

If you are a healthcare professional, especially a doctor or a nurse, you may prefer to read more advanced resources such as textbooks for pediatricians and neonatologists. My favorite textbook for neonatologists was written by Fanaroff and Martin.

If you are a person who gets depressed or easily scared while reading about potentially adverse outcomes, you may want to ask your partner or friend to read the book first before deciding to do so yourself. I remember one mother, whom I met during my career, who refused to see her baby for several days after birth. She had carefully preplanned her natural in-water delivery and her care for the baby after birth. However, she ended up having an emergency Cesarean section, and the baby needed resuscitation and intensive care using a ventilator. The reality turned out to be so far from the mother's dreams that she did not want to face it. She explained that she did not want to see her baby on a ventilator, with all the monitors, intravenous (IV) catheters, and tubes. She only went to see her baby several days later when it looked strong and healthy. Everybody reacts very differently to trauma, and we need to respect that and be empathetic.

It is essential to understand that, for many parents, experience of having a child in a NICU may trigger post-traumatic stress disorder (PTSD). All healthcare providers, family members, and friends should be on the lookout for any symptoms of mental ill health in parents of premature babies. We can support these parents in many ways: let's take care of their other children so that they can spend more time in the NICU; let's cook for them; let's call them often to ask how they are doing. However, do not necessarily ask them how their newborn is doing unless they volunteer that information—having them repeat the same sad news to everybody is not a good idea. I advise parents to designate one trusted person to communicate between them and the other friends and family members regarding the condition of the baby in the unit.

I sincerely believe that your NICU journey will be more comfortable and less confusing thanks to my book, and I wish you the best possible health outcome for your treasured baby.

M. Wisniewski

CHAPTER 2

How to use this book?

I am a big proponent of the adult learning theory. This theory says that adults are independent learners and enjoy the learning process most when they can decide for themselves what and how to study. I strongly encourage you to do exactly that with this book. In the next few paragraphs, I will give you more details regarding what topics are covered in each chapter.

One can assign the content of this book to one of four groups of topics:

Group 1: General information (Chapters 1–5, 20)

In these chapters, I introduce you to the neonatal intensive care unit (NICU), describe the people who work there and also the equipment. I talk about prematurity and common conditions affecting premature babies in the NICU, and I describe typical diagnostic and therapeutic procedures used to treat babies receiving intensive care.

Group 2: Common problems and therapies in the neonatal intensive care unit (Chapters 6–10, 12, 18, 20)

In these chapters, I focus specifically on the conditions that affect almost all premature babies born before 32 weeks. Problems such as respiratory distress syndrome, apnea, feeding issues, newborn jaundice, and infections belong to this category.

Group 3: Complications of prematurity (Chapters 11, 13–19)

Not all premature babies develop severe complications of prematurity, but we do monitor them all for that possibility. Serious complications of prematurity such as bronchopulmonary dysplasia, necrotizing enterocolitis, patent ductus arteriosus, retinopathy of prematurity, intraventricular hemorrhage, and anemias belong in this group.

Group 4: Other topics (Chapters 21–24)

In Chapter 21, I talk at length about outcomes for premature babies, particularly survival rates and developmental outcomes after discharge home. Chapter 22 covers congenital anomalies and genetic syndromes. These topics are not specific to premature babies. However, if your baby is affected, it will be useful to read it. Chapters 23 and 24 deal with issues related to discharge home and care needed afterwards.

The order in which you want to read different chapters may depend on your specific situation. If you are still pregnant but worried that you might have a premature baby, just read the chapters in Group 1. They will familiarize you with the NICU, prematurity, and common conditions affecting premature babies. If your baby is already born, but less than 1 to 2 weeks old, read the chapters in Groups 1 and 2 first.

If your little one is in a NICU and was born more than 1 month ago, you will probably be interested in learning about complications of prematurity. You will find this information in the chapters from Group 3.

While writing this book, I deviated on purpose from the typical style often used in "books for parents." I intentionally introduced more medical information than is customary, and I gave names of reference articles from which I cited statistical data. The latter part is vital to me. In my opinion, doctors regularly underestimate the drive for more information that their patients and families have. By providing you with references, I wanted to encourage you to expand your knowledge using credible scientific articles. I know that some readers will not stop with my book: they will want to read more and more from other available resources.

CHAPTER 3

I have a premature baby—what to do now?

I f you have just given birth to a premature baby, you may be asking what you should do now. That is a great question. Nobody and nothing could prepare you for such an eventuality unless you had previously had another premature baby. Even in such a case, you are probably in a state of disbelief, saying: "Oh, not again!" Often, after the birth of a premature baby, I see parents who seem a little bit lost and not knowing what to do. So I want to prepare you a little for what is to come.

Let's discuss a few things—in no particular order—that you should consider doing if you have just become a parent of a premature baby.

Take a deep breath

If you are reading this book, it probably means that your baby is alive, and that is a big thing! You gave life to somebody, and you should be proud of yourself. I know it is difficult for you, but you have to preserve your strength for a long fight. It will help if you are ready for it emotionally and physically. Depending on the degree of prematurity, your baby may need to stay in the hospital for any time from weeks to several months and, in some cases, even for a year or longer.

Psychologists compare being a parent of a premature baby with being a soldier on a battlefield. Such parents are at significant risk of developing post-traumatic stress disorder (PTSD) or depression. Nowadays, staff in some larger neonatal intensive care units (NICUs) are aware of that, and involve psychologists and social workers to check on parents of a premature baby. These professionals can provide help when needed. Family members, friends, doctors, and nurses also need to be on the lookout for any signs of postpartum depression in mothers and to intervene if warranted.

Check if the hospital where your baby is receiving medical care is the right or best place for your baby

First, when deciding whether to leave your premature baby in the current hospital, you need to consider your insurance plan.

If you have medical insurance other than Medicaid (relates to US market only), you probably know that some hospitals are—and some are not—in the so-called "network." Your payments may vary significantly depending on where your baby is hospitalized. If this is important to you, talk to your insurance company and hospital case management worker to sort it out. The insurance company may agree to cover all the services for your baby even if it is not an "in-network" hospital. However, it is always better to check it as early as possible to avoid unexpected hospital bills. Sadly, hospital charges for the care of premature babies can run into hundreds of thousands of dollars.

Second, you should find out whether your baby's hospital is the right one from the medical and quality point of view. In neonatal care, NICU and nurseries receive a level of care designation, as follows:

Level 3 and 4 NICUs can provide appropriate care to pretty much all types of babies at different gestational ages and with all kinds of complications. Most big level 3 and 4 NICUs will be staffed by neonatologists always on site. If it is important to you that there is always a neonatologist available to your baby at a moment's notice, you should ask about this.

A level 2 Nursery typically provides care to babies born at 32 weeks of gestational age or more, and without severe or prolonged respiratory problems. There will be considerable variability in how these level 2 units are staffed. Some will have neonatologists; others will have nurse practitioners or pediatricians working there. If a neonatologist is not always available on site, he or she will be always available by phone to be consulted on more complicated cases.

A level 1 Nursery is a place where we take care of healthy term newborn babies. In most cases, pediatricians or family practice doctors provide care to babies staying in level 1 nurseries.

You should ask your doctor whether the NICU, where your baby is being treated, is the right and best place for them to be now. Sometimes your baby will need a transfer to another institution for further care. Obviously, in all situations, one has to consider the benefits and risks for your baby before deciding on a transfer to another hospital.

Find out who your baby's doctor and primary nurse are

In most hospitals, there will be numerous doctors who will be seeing and taking care of your baby, such as:

- residents (doctors in training);
- fellows (these are sub-specialty doctors in training);
- pediatric hospitalists (pediatricians who provide care in the hospital);
- neonatologists (pediatricians with additional training in the care of newborns and premature babies);
- cardiologists;

- surgeons; and
- many others.

Usually, there will be one doctor with a specialization in neonatology—who will be on service for a week or a month—and who will be responsible for managing the medical care of your baby. You should definitely know who that person is.

After birth, once your baby's condition is stabilized, a doctor will come to your bedside and give you all the initial information. They will tell you in general terms how sick your baby is at the moment and what to expect in the next few hours and days. Usually, discussions about long-term outcomes are left for later: until the doctors have a better idea of how your baby is doing and you have had a chance to recover from the stressful experience of delivering a premature baby. You can ask how often you will receive updates and whom you can contact if you would like to check on your baby. Always, the fastest and easiest way of following your baby's progress is knowing who their nurse is during each shift and then contacting that person directly.

Plan to spend time with your baby at their bedside

You will want to be in the hospital at your baby's bedside and holding your baby as much as you can. But you will have to consider different factors such as your family situation (other children and pets) and available family and friends who can potentially help you at home.

Your job situation may influence your decisions. For most employed people, it is difficult to take extended time off work. If you have limited time off that you can take, the smart thing usually is to take some time off initially so that you can be with your baby during the first days or week when they are in their most critical condition. Save the rest of the time available to you for when your baby is closer to being discharged home. That way, you will have time to learn how to take care of your baby's needs before they leave the NICU. Some people will face a difficult decision, provided they can afford it, if it makes sense for them to quit their job altogether.

Consider providing breast milk for your baby

Breast milk is by far the best and most valuable medication that your premature baby can receive. Please take note that I called breast milk a "medication". I've done that on purpose. Breast milk is particularly critical for extremely premature babies and micro-preemies. If your baby was born before 32 weeks of gestational age, it is unlikely that you will be able to put your baby to the breast in the first few days after birth. However, it will help if you start pumping breast milk as soon as you can. Because your body went through very different adjustments compared with delivery at full term, it does not know that your baby needs milk. You need to pump milk regularly, every 2 to 3 hours, so that your body gets used to it and you start producing milk naturally.

It may be very helpful for your milk supply if you do "kangaroo care" (also known as "skin-to-skin care" (see Chapter 7), provided your baby can tolerate that. You would be surprised that very tiny babies, even when they are sick, tend to tolerate kangaroo care pretty well. Often, such a baby is more stable in your arms than when they are placed alone in an "isolette" (or "incubator").

Learn as much as you can about prematurity and the conditions associated with it

Knowledge about the health issues affecting you or your family members is frequently under-appreciated. You need to fully understand what is going on with your baby at all times. Your knowledge will help you make better decisions about their care when discussing different options with their doctors.

There are many resources available from which you can learn more about prematurity. In addition to this book, you can expand your knowledge by visiting the websites of the following organizations:

1. March of Dimes: A charitable organization that provides education, advocacy, and research funding aimed at prenatal health, congenital disabilities, and genetics: https://www.marchofdimes.org
2. WebMD: An American corporation that publishes online news and information about human health and well-being: https://www.webmd.com
3. National Institute of Health: A government organization focusing on research and education: https://www.nih.gov
4. Centers for Disease Control and Prevention: A government agency providing reliable information about various health topics: https://www.cdc.gov

CHAPTER 4

Prematurity— background Information

I n this chapter, I will first discuss the definition of prematurity and the different terms used to describe premature babies. Then I will talk about common medical conditions associated with prematurity and how we treat them. The term "prematurity" defines a baby either born before 37 weeks of gestational age or more than three weeks earlier than its due date. Another way of defining it is that the premature baby is born at fewer than 259 days after the onset of the mother's last menstrual period. There are also many qualifying terms used to describe the severity of prematurity but definitions of these are not always precise. I will talk about the most frequently used ones here:

Mild prematurity: When a baby is born at a gestational age of more than 32 weeks but fewer than 37 weeks. Birth weight is usually above 1,500 grams.

Moderate prematurity: When a baby is born between 28 weeks and 32 weeks of gestational age. Birth weight is usually between 1,000 and 1,500 grams.

Extreme prematurity: When a baby is born at fewer than 28 weeks of gestational age and with a birth weight below 1,000 grams.

Also, with the increasing survival of tiny babies, some people use the term "*micro-preemie*." This is generally used to describe babies born at fewer than 26 weeks of gestational age and with a birth weight below 800 grams.

In addition to terms describing the degree of prematurity, doctors use qualifiers to give information regarding a baby's weight in relation to expected weights for the particular gestational age group. After birth, we plot the baby's birth weight on a growth chart to find out whether it is AGA, SGA, or LGA.

"AGA" means "appropriate weight for gestational age" and the term is assigned to a baby when their weight is between the 10th and 90th percentile on the growth chart. In other words, 10% of all babies born at the same age as the AGA baby will have a weight below the 10th percentile and will be called "SGA" or "small for gestational age", 80% of the babies will have birth weights between the 10th and 90th percentile and will be called AGA, and 10% of babies will have weights above the 90th percentile and will be called "LGA" or "large for gestational age." Assigning an SGA, AGA, or LGA classification to a baby's weight helps anticipate specific problems that are more common to a particular group of babies. For example, for the same gestational age, SGA babies tend to have less severe breathing problems, but they will have more issues with regulation of their body temperature, glucose levels, and proper brain development.

Another term that you may hear used to describe your baby is "IUGR". This stands for "intrauterine growth restriction." It is a diagnosis made by an obstetrician based on several ultrasound examinations performed during pregnancy. It means that the baby's weight does not follow the initially assigned percentile rank. For example, at 12 weeks, the fetus weight was at the 50th percentile for its gestational age; at 15 weeks, it was at the 30th percentile; and at birth at 28 weeks it was at the 20th percentile. Whenever we see such a pattern of weight falling off the initially assigned percentile rank, we talk about the baby or fetus not fulfilling its initial growth potential. IUGR may be caused by maternal medical conditions, problems with the placenta, or conditions originating in the baby.

How common is premature birth?

In 2017 in the USA, we had 3.8 million live births. Out of those, 10% were born prematurely—that is, about 380,000 premature babies in a year. A staggering number! There is a substantial racial disparity in rates of prematurity. Only 9% of white non-Hispanic babies are born prematurely, and almost 14% of black babies are premature at birth. The exact explanation for this disparity is still unknown. Only 0.67% of all babies are born before 28 weeks of gestational age. However, this percentage still constitutes a large number of infants. Approximately 26,000 babies across the whole country are born at fewer than 28 weeks.

What are the causes of premature birth?

Whenever I speak to parents of a premature baby for the first time, I am almost always asked what caused it. Did they do something wrong? I quickly reassure them that it is nobody's fault and, most importantly, it is not the mother's fault. In 50% of cases, pregnant mothers go into preterm labor spontaneously. In 40%, they have preterm rupture of the membranes that results in the birth of a premature baby. In 10% of cases, there are maternal medical indications to deliver the baby early. There are multiple risk factors cited in the literature that are associated with preterm delivery. These can be divided into four categories: demographic factors, behavioral factors, maternal medical conditions, and pregnancy complications:

Among demographic factors, we know that women who are black, younger than 17 or older than 35, less educated, or from lower socio-economic status have higher rates of premature births.

Among behavioral factors, poor nutritional status, low body mass index, smoking, substance abuse, lack of prenatal care, and stress contribute to higher rates of premature labor.

Maternal medical conditions, such as uterine or cervical malformations, myomas, high blood pressure, and diabetes are associated with higher rates of premature births.

Pregnancy characteristics, such as twins or triplets, an increased or decreased amount of amniotic fluid, vaginal bleeding, low body mass index, fetal anomalies, abdominal surgery, and infections are known to be associated with higher rates of premature births.

I want to emphasize that these associations do not mean a cause–effect relationship. If you are pregnant and have one or even several risk factors associated with premature delivery, you should not panic. A smart thing to do is to ensure that you are receiving prenatal care from doctors who are familiar with taking care of high-risk pregnancy and can start appropriate monitoring to use preventive measures if needed.

How are premature babies cared for?

Every premature baby has *a unique set of problems and challenges* that the doctors need to address. However, it would be safe to say that almost all babies born before 32 weeks of gestational age will be treated using all the treatment modalities listed below. I will explain "why" and "how" about each one.

Standard therapies used to care for premature babies in the neonatal intensive care unit (NICU) are as follows:

- Provision of a neutral thermal environment.
- Tube feedings and intravenous (IV) fluids.
- Respiratory support.
- Medications: surfactant, antibiotics, caffeine, Indomethacin, or Ibuprofen.

- Routine measures such as Hepatitis B vaccine, Vitamin K, and Erythromycin eye ointment.

Provision of a neutral thermal environment

Most premature babies are unable to maintain normal body temperature after birth. Many times, this problem—along with poor feeding—is the last one that gets resolved before a baby can go home. It is common that the baby has gained enough weight, can eat well, and has resolved all breathing problems, but still needs to be in an isolette (or "incubator") to stay warm.

Premature babies get cold because of:

1. small body weight and a thin layer of skin and fat;
2. an immature brain that is unable to regulate temperature well;
3. an inadequate amount of energy sources in the body; and
4. metabolic immaturity

Premature babies who have body temperature problems and are staying in the NICU will be placed in an isolette or on a *radiant warmer bed*. The latter is a small table with a mattress on it and a heat lamp above. We use it right after delivery and during the first few hours of life for stabilization and to perform procedures. An isolette is a more permanent solution: it is a plastic box into which we blow warmed and humidified air. The amount of heat is regulated automatically by a computer and adjusted to the baby's needs. Babies are kept in isolettes until they are ready to come out to an open crib, usually close to their discharge home.

Feedings and fluids

The feeding process requires three separate physiological functions to be developed and coordinated well: sucking, swallowing, and breathing. Maturation of feeding skills usually starts at around 32 to 34 weeks of gestational age and is sometimes not even completed until 38 weeks of corrected gestational age. When a premature baby is very sick, we can provide fluids and all necessary nutrients intravenously. If we expect that the baby will need IV nutrition for a long time, we insert special types of IV catheters called "central lines." Veins in babies are very tiny and maintaining regular IV access beyond several days is challenging, if not impossible—thus the need for central lines.

As soon as premature babies are stable, they are started on tube feedings. These are also called "gavage" or "NG/OG" feedings. A nurse inserts a small, flexible, plastic tube directly into the stomach through the nose or mouth. Then she connects a syringe with breast milk or formula and the milk is delivered directly into the baby's stomach. Once the baby is around 32 weeks of gestational age and is showing interest in oral feedings, a nurse will try bottle feeding while continuing to give the remaining milk through the tube. Eventually, virtually all newborns learn how to eat by mouth, but for some it will be a very long process.

Respiratory support

The vast majority of premature babies develop breathing problems after birth for which they need to be treated. They may suffer from different respiratory problems: respiratory distress syndrome (RDS, see Chapter 8), bronchopulmonary dysplasia (BPD, see Chapter 11), transient tachypnea of newborns, or pneumonia. In general, the type of respiratory support does not depend on the particular disease—rather, it depends on the severity of the respiratory problem.

Many babies with breathing problems need supplementary oxygen to maintain appropriate oxygenation levels. Room air has 21% oxygen. However, if required by the baby, we can provide up to 100% oxygen. Extra oxygen can be provided using an oxyhood, nasal cannulas, continuous positive airway pressure (CPAP) devices, or ventilators:

An oxyhood: This is a plastic box that surrounds the baby's head. One can blow air with supplementary oxygen into it to increase the availability of oxygen to the baby. It is used very rarely for premature babies.

A nasal cannula: This is plastic tubing that is placed in a baby's nose. It provides an increased flow of the air–oxygen mixture. It is used only for very mild respiratory diseases.

A CPAP device: This delivers a flow of the air–oxygen mixture with the addition of extra airway pressure during the expiratory phase of breathing effort. While on CPAP, the baby is still breathing entirely on its own. This technique is used for moderately sick babies.

A ventilator or "breathing machine": This is used for the most severely sick newborns. It can support the baby's breathing efforts or provide all external breaths for the baby who is not breathing.

Medications

We don't use many medicines to treat premature babies. This is because the main reason why premature babies are sick is their physiologic immaturity. There is no medication capable of speeding up the maturity of all organs in a baby. Therefore, during their NICU stay, doctors mainly support their maturation processes by maintaining all physiologic functions—we do not treat any particular sickness per se.

However, I describe below a few medications that we do use in NICUs.

Antibiotics (Ampicillin and Gentamicin)

Infection in a mother may be a cause of premature delivery and, consequently, the baby may be infected. It is common practice to treat sick premature babies after birth with antibiotics (most commonly with Ampicillin and Gentamicin) while waiting for blood test results. These will tell us if the baby has an infection or not. Because many babies undergo invasive procedures, they are at risk for complications such as infections. Any sudden deterioration of the general condition in a baby may be the first sign of such. Hospital-acquired infections are always treated with antibiotics.

Caffeine

Most premature babies born before 32 weeks of gestational age will develop apnea of prematurity. Apnea is a condition where the baby "forgets" to breathe for 10 to 20 seconds. Caffeine, which is a chemical substance also found in tea and coffee, is the drug of choice to treat apnea of prematurity.

Surfactant

Respiratory distress syndrome (RDS) is the most common respiratory disease in babies born before 32 weeks of gestational age. This condition is due to anatomic and chemical immaturity of the lungs. In this disease, lungs lack a chemical substance called "surfactant," which prevents distal portions of the lungs from collapsing. Fortunately, scientists are able to extract surfactant from animals and synthesize it in a lab. We can administer it to sick newborn babies with RDS. To do so, we have to put a breathing tube into the windpipe. We inject surfactant via that tube directly into the baby's lungs. After the administration of the surfactant, babies are usually placed on a CPAP device or ventilator.

Indometacin, Ibuprofen or Acetaminophen for treatment of patent ductus arteriosus (see <u>Chapter 14</u>)

The cardiovascular system of the fetus differs from that of newborn babies. Immediately after birth, specific changes should take place in the circulatory system of the baby. In some premature babies, those processes do not occur and some blood vessels, which should stop functioning and close, still function and create problems for the baby. One of these conditions is called "patent ductus arteriosus" (PDA).

PDA may contribute to blood pressure or breathing problems in a baby. Therefore, sometimes, it needs to be treated. We can do this medically with Indomethacin, Ibuprofen, or Acetaminophen. If the baby does not respond favorably to the medication, surgery may also be an option.

Phototherapy (see <u>Chapter 10</u>)

Jaundice or hyperbilirubinemia is a condition in which the baby presents with a yellow skin color. It is probably the most common pathology occurring in both full-term and premature babies. Some babies who need treatment will be started on phototherapy. Phototherapy is a light therapy that changes the properties of the bilirubin (a culprit in jaundice disease) in the baby's skin, allowing for its faster excretion from the body. It therefore protects the baby's brain from the harming effects of bilirubin.

Routine measures (see <u>Chapter 6</u>)

Just because a baby is born prematurely does not mean we can forgo all preventive measures offered to full-term babies. Depending on their gestational age and birth weight, the following procedures will be given to all premature babies:

- Vitamin K after birth to prevent bleeding.
- Hepatitis B vaccine to prevent Hepatitis B viral disease.
- Two months' vaccinations if the baby is still in the NICU.
- Erythromycin ointment right after birth to prevent gonococcal infection in the baby's eyes.
- A "car seat test" before discharge home.
- A hearing test before discharge home.

In this chapter, I have given you only an overview of different therapies used in the NICU. In later chapters, I will expand on many specific problems encountered in premature babies and talk about their treatments in more detail.

CHAPTER 5

Neonatal intensive care units

I n this chapter, I will talk about the environment within the neonatal intensive care unit (NICU). I will describe what you are likely to encounter in the unit during your baby's stay. For most family members, often stressed out, coming to a NICU for the first time is an overwhelming experience. Parents have to face a new place with many unknown people and plenty of strange-looking pieces of equipment. The goal of this chapter is to ease those anxieties.

The NICU is the place where we care for the sickest newborn babies. Usually, the full name is reserved for the type of nursery where the highest level of care can be provided. At the minimum, that includes cardiorespiratory monitoring (in other words, heart and respiratory rate monitoring) and respiratory support equipment such as ventilators and continuous positive airway pressure (CPAP) machines.

Most commonly, in the USA, NICUs are run by pediatric sub-specialists called "neonatologists." In rare situations, particularly outside the USA, pediatric intensivists or pediatric anesthesiologists may be in charge of patients in these units.

"ICN" stands for intermediate care nursery. It is a place where we take care of less severely sick newborn babies. Usually, babies located in an ICN won't have any life-threatening conditions and won't need ventilatory support any more, but they will still need monitoring and medical care. ICNs are units that are in between a NICU and a regular nursery. Sometimes, an ICN is also called a "step-down unit," which means that patients there will be less sick than those in a NICU.

In some areas, people use the term "SCN" (special care nursery) to describe hospital wards where sick newborn babies are cared for. However, SCN is not often used and it is a less specific term than NICU or ICN. Occasionally, SCN is used to indicate a level 2 nursery (see explanations below about levels of care).

"Nursery" may mean a place where any type of newborn (both healthy and sick) are located. In most hospitals, the term is used to describe a ward with only healthy full-term or near full-term babies.

What does "the NICU level of care" mean in newborn medicine?

Parents should pay particular attention to the designated level of care in the unit where their baby is receiving treatment. In the USA and many Western countries, hospitals receive—or assign to themselves—the designated level of care. It will be based on available personnel, equipment, clinical capabilities, and experience. Some US states have strict criteria regarding this matter and others are more relaxed about it. The American Academy of Pediatrics developed guidelines as to how to decide on the levels of neonatal care. However, those guidelines are not strictly followed by all states.

Nurseries may receive a level designation ranging from 1 to 4, with level 1 being the lowest and level 4 being the highest level of care possible.

Nursery level 1

A level 1 nursery typically provides care for stable term new-born infants and for premature babies born at 35 weeks or later who also remain physiologically stable. Babies who do not meet these criteria need to be stabilized and transferred to a facility with a higher level of care. Usually, a level 1 nursery is staffed by pediatricians, family physicians, and nurse practitioners. It would be rare for a neonatologist to practice at such a place. However, a neonatologist may be available for consultations over the phone.

Nursery level 2

A level 2 nursery, also called an "SCN" by some, will have all the capabilities of a level 1 nursery and will also be able to provide care for:

- babies born at 32 weeks or more of gestational age or with a weight of more than 1,500 grams;
- babies who have "graduated" from a level 3 NICU; and
- babies who require mechanical ventilation or CPAP for no more than 24 hours.

Newborns who do not meet the criteria for level 2, and need more complex care, will have to be transferred to a level 3 or level 4 NICU.

Level 2 nurseries can be staffed by pediatric hospitalists, neonatal nurse practitioners, and neonatologists.

Nursery level 3

A level 3 nursery, also called a "NICU", is capable of providing continuous life support for all kinds of premature and term babies without a lower limit in gestational age. They will treat babies starting from 22 or 23 weeks of gestational age (the usual limit of viability).

It is expected that a level 3 NICU will be staffed by neonatologists and have other pediatric sub-specialists available.

Nursery level 4

A level 4 nursery is called a "regional neonatal intensive care unit". In addition to neonatologists, this type of NICU will be staffed by all pediatric sub-specialists, even including pediatric surgical sub-specialists, and will be able to treat complicated congenital heart defects as well as other congenital and genetic abnormalities. A level 4 NICU should have continuous transport availability and be actively involved in outreach education at other institutions.

Ideally, if you are at risk of having a very premature baby (born below 32 weeks of gestational age), you should deliver your baby at a level 3 hospital, but that is not always the case. I have heard of some future parents who, when knowing that they were at risk of having a premature baby, would relocate temporarily to be close to their chosen level 3 hospital until their baby was born. On the other hand, I have met parents who have resisted recommended transfer of their baby to a higher level of care unit because of the distance that they would need to travel while visiting. I understand that each family has a unique situation, and we have to respect that. Still, experience and the level of care given to your baby in the nursery are very important, so sometimes the transfer of your baby to another institution is in their best interest.

Who are the people working in the NICU?

Neonatologists: These are physicians who specialize in the care of newborn babies. After graduating from medical school, they would have done three years of pediatric residency training and later an additional three years of fellowship in neonatology (in the USA—it may be different in other countries). These physicians have the highest level of training in newborn medicine, allowing them to take care of extremely sick and premature babies.

Frequently, they also attend high-risk deliveries and provide consultations to pediatricians who may have questions regarding their patients, such as "normal" regular full-term newborns. If you are curious about your physician's training and certification (in the USA), you can check it on the American Board of Pediatrics' website (https://www.abp.org). You can practice this by entering my name there: "Wlodzimierz Wisniewski."

Neonatal nurse practitioners (NNPs): An NNP is sometimes called a "mid-level healthcare provider." They are people who first used to work as nurses in the NICU and, later on, decided to obtain additional training in neonatology so that they could provide more independent care to newborn babies in all kinds of settings. They usually hold Master's degrees or, recently, even doctorate degrees. They are treasured members of the NICU team and, together with neonatologists, provide care for all sick newborn babies. In complex situations, NNPs need to obtain a consultation from a neonatologist because frequently they work under neonatologists' supervision.

Respiratory therapists (RTs): These are trained in the use of different devices to support breathing and oxygenation in a patient. These devices include ventilators (also called "breathing machines"), CPAP devices, face masks, nasal cannulas, and oxygen tents. RTs know how to set up equipment for use, what adjustments in settings should be made in different situations, and how to clear secretions from the airway in a baby. They are essential members of the NICU team, particularly during the first days of life of fragile newborn babies who need treatment for severe respiratory distress symptoms.

Pharmacy doctors (PharmDs): These are professionals trained in the use of various medicines. They are needed in NICUs because premature babies have a very different and unique physiology. Responses of newborn babies to pharmaceuticals differ from those of adult patients or even from those of children. Also, frequent use of intravenous (IV) nutrition called "hyperalimentation" necessitates the presence of PharmDs because they are the experts in this area.

Registered nurses (RNs): These are skilled caretakers who spend the most time with the babies. In my humble opinion, they are *the most important* team members in the NICU. Usually, they take care of 1 to 4 babies, depending on the babies' acuity levels. They know your baby best. I do not know any good neonatologist who would not seriously consider a concern brought to their attention by an experienced RN. Often, RNs are the first to notice that a baby is getting into trouble and needs extra attention, such as a diagnostic test or treatment. To say that they are the best advocates and guardian angels for your baby, when you are not present at your baby's bedside, would not be an overstatement.

Pediatric sub-specialists such as cardiologists, pulmonologists, ID specialists, and pediatric surgeons: These people are pediatricians with extra training in their sub-specialty. They are often called by neonatologists to give their expertise regarding a particular problem that your baby may be having. They examine your baby when asked and discuss with neonatologists what the best course of action is to tackle the problem. Depending on the issue, they may talk to you directly to provide specific information regarding your baby's problems with their heart, lungs, kidney, or brain.

Occupational and physical therapists (OTs/PTs) evaluate and stimulate appropriate development of motor and feeding skills in your baby. Often they are also involved in the care of your baby after discharge. They participate in developmental assessments and early intervention programs aimed to ensure the proper motor and intellectual development of your baby after discharge home.

It is only natural to see a lot of students in a NICU. Doctors who practice where your baby is staying are probably treating many very sick babies. Therefore, there will be many different people who will be learning the difficult craft of medicine from them. These may be medical, nursing, respiratory therapy, and PharmD students, as well as medical residents and fellows:

Medical residents are young doctors who have graduated from medical school and are in training in their chosen specialty.

Fellows are physicians who have already received one broader specialty training, and are now learning in a more specialized area—for example, pediatricians who want to become neonatologists.

I know it may be overwhelming to see so many people around your baby. Hearing their opinions or statements will be confusing. On the surface, it may seem that when they give you information they contradict each other and cause you frustration and anxiety. My best advice is to allow students and younger doctors to learn but, whenever it is too much for you, ask for privacy. Any time you are not sure what's going on with your baby, ask to talk to their nurse and the neonatologists in charge.

Equipment in the neonatal intensive care unit

When you come to a NICU for the first time, you will see many pieces of equipment used to care for babies.

After birth, your baby will be placed on a *radiant warmer bed*. This is a table with a heat lamp above it to keep babies warm. The advantage of this table-bed is that it provides easy access to your baby from 3 to 4 sides. That way, during critical moments, several people can treat your baby at the same time. After all the procedures are done, and your baby is stable, the staff will put your baby in an isolette (incubator). Babies are not kept on radiant warmer beds for a long time because this would expose them to frequently changing environmental temperatures, drafts, and noise, and they also tend to lose a lot of water through evaporation from their immature skin.

The isolette is a plastic box with double walls that provides a controlled environment for your baby. It allows doctors to continuously regulate the air temperature and humidity inside the box to meet your baby's individual needs.

Many level 3 and 4 units have at their disposal a hybrid bed solution called a "giraffe incubator." This is an incubator that allows a quick elevation of the roof and pulling down of the side walls to transform it into a radiant warmer bed, and vice versa, without the need to move the baby from one place to another.

Once your baby grows bigger and stronger, usually above 3 to 4 pounds of body weight (1.8 kg), they will be placed in an *open crib*. This will occur in preparation for the future discharge home and is always a good sign. It means that your baby can regulate their body temperature, just dressed in clothes for newborns and covered with a blanket without additional external heat sources.

What types of monitors are used in the unit?

All premature babies who are admitted to an NICU are continuously monitored until their discharge home. Monitors can measure heart rate, respiratory rate, blood pressure, and amount of oxygen attached to the hemoglobin (called "oxygen saturation"). Monitors gather all that information from the baby after leads are placed on the baby's body, usually on the chest, abdomen, and extremities. Leads need to be made of very soft materials to avoid skin irritation. We try to change the positioning of the leads frequently to allow for skin recovery, especially in babies who have very immature and sensitive skin.

Respiratory support in the unit

Pretty much all very premature babies require some kind of respiratory support. Depending on the severity of respiratory problems and degree of recovery during hospitalization, you may see your baby first on a ventilator, then a CPAP machine, a high flow cannula, and finally on a low flow cannula.

A ventilator, sometimes called a *"respirator"* or *"breathing machine,"* is a device that provides artificial or external breathing for your baby. First, we insert a small plastic breathing tube called an "ET tube" through the mouth into the windpipe. Then, we connect the tube to the breathing machine. The breathing machine provides breathing for the baby when needed, leading to adequate expansion, aeration, and oxygenation of the lungs. Modern breathing machines contain intelligent sensors and computer software that can decide when a baby can be allowed to breathe on its own and when to intervene by adding external airflow and pressure. Most of the time, sick babies somehow know that they need this support and tolerate being supported by the machines very well.

A CPAP device is a less aggressive form of respiratory support. A baby placed on CPAP has a special nasal apparatus inside or around the nose that is connected to a CPAP device. They have to be able to breathe on their own while on CPAP because a simple CPAP machine does not provide external breaths. A CPAP device only provides additional pressure and a mixture of air with supplementary oxygen into the baby's airways. With CPAP machines, we can control the amount of oxygen getting to the baby's lungs and airway pressure at the end of expiration. Many neonatologists try to limit a baby's exposure to ventilators. Hence they have invented a hybrid CPAP machine that can provide some external breaths. This newer technique is called "non-invasive positive pressure ventilation."

High flow nasal cannulas are used for babies who have already recovered from acute respiratory disease after birth and do not need ventilators any more, or who are less sick but still require some respiratory support. The high flow cannula device provides airflow with supplementary oxygen via a small cannula placed in the baby's nose. Airflows provided range from 3 to 5 liters per minute.

A low flow cannula is used in babies who do not have severe respiratory problems any more and just need a little bit of extra oxygen for breathing to maintain proper oxygenation levels in their blood. Sometimes babies with chronic lung disease, who need oxygen for breathing but otherwise are ready for home, are sent home with low flow cannulas. These low flow cannulas provide no more than 1 to 2 liters per minute of flow into the baby's nose with additional oxygen whenever needed.

Other types of equipment in the NICU are as follows:

IV fluid pumps and *medication syringe pumps* are electronic devices that can infuse medications and nutritional fluids at carefully measured rates. During the first weeks and months of life, your baby will be receiving many medications and various IV fluids. IV pumps are used to deliver the exact amount of whatever the doctors prescribed. Pumps may be attached to poles next to an isolette, they may be placed on top of the isolette, or they may be attached to parts of the isolette with special screws. Often one baby will be receiving medications and fluids from 3 or 4 pumps simultaneously.

Phototherapy lamps are used to treat jaundice (yellow skin is a symptom) in newborn babies. Premature babies are likely to develop jaundice that will need phototherapy treatment. Phototherapy can be provided using overhead bank lamps, spot lamps that are integrated with the baby's isolette, or bili blankets. A "bili blanket" has numerous tiny bulbs built into it. One can place this under the baby or wrap it around the baby. Phototherapy uses specific light wavelengths shined onto the baby's skin to decrease the severity of jaundice. I will talk more about this particular problem in Chapter 10.

CHAPTER 6

"Normal routine" newborn care

There is nothing "normal" and "routine" about the medical care we provide for premature babies. Still, certain procedures are the same for both preterm and term newborns. This chapter will focus on evaluations and procedures that newborn babies undergo right after birth, or before they go home, regardless of their gestational age at birth. Before babies are discharged home, we do a lot to ensure their well-being. We do things to promote their good health and to detect whether they have any medical conditions that require immediate treatment or follow-up. I will concentrate here on the care provided in the USA. Sometimes, other doctors, institutions, and countries may be doing things differently.

Birth of the baby

Personally, I call the first 10 minutes after birth "the 10 happy minutes." It is one of the few situations in our life when we see a baby loudly and vigorously crying, and everybody else in the room smiling and overwhelmed with joy. It is that way because this vigorous cry—if it occurs—is a sign of life and good health. The first thing to do to a baby after birth is to clamp and cut the umbilical cord. Usually, the father will have the opportunity to do that. Then the nurse or somebody else will assign Apgar scores (see below), take the baby's weight, count their respiratory and heart rates, and measure their body temperature.

If the baby is healthy and close to full term, we may just give them to the mother as soon as the umbilical cord has been cut. Holding the baby skin to skin will promote mother–baby bonding and establish a better breastfeeding routine. Unfortunately, for many premature babies, that may not be possible. Premature babies with respiratory problems are handed quickly to the neonatal team for stabilization and treatment.

Cutting the umbilical cord

The umbilical cord is like a "lifeline." It is a connection between the fetus and the mother through which delivery of nutrients, hormones, growth factors, and oxygen occurs. After the baby is born, this connection will be interrupted, and part of the umbilical cord on the baby's side needs to be securely clamped so that they do not lose any blood. In the past few decades, the umbilical cord would have been clamped soon after the baby was born. Nowadays, it is suggested to extend the time between birth and the clamping of the cord. We believe that the baby may benefit by acquiring additional blood from the placenta if clamping is delayed until 1 to 3 minutes after birth. Approach to umbilical cord clamping differs among doctors and institutions. Therefore, if you have not delivered your baby yet, you may want to discuss this with your obstetrician. Also, delay in umbilical cord clamping may not be possible if the newborn requires immediate resuscitation.

Assigning the Apgar score

Apgar scoring is a method of assessing a newborn baby's well-being after birth. It was developed by Dr Virginia Apgar in 1952 and widely accepted by nurseries as a reproducible and straightforward tool with which to make an initial assessment.

Table 6.1

Sign	0 points	1 point	2 points
Heart rate (HR)	No heart rate at all	HR <100/min	HR >100/min
Respiratory effort	No respirations	Slow, irregular	Regular, strong
Muscle tone	Flaccid	Limbs flexed	Moving well
Reflex to stimulus	No reaction	Grimace	Strong reaction
Skin color	Pale, grey all over	Peripheral cyanosis	Pink all over

Today, all nurseries assign Apgar scores at 1, 5, and 10 minutes after birth. It is done in five categories. For each element of the assessment, we can assign a value of 0, 1, or 2. We add up numerical values in each category and record the final score. An Apgar score of 0 means that the baby was born without any signs of life. An Apgar score of 10 is the best one can achieve, meaning that the baby was very vigorous, spontaneously breathing without any difficulty, had normal muscle tone, and was well oxygenated.

The initial purpose of the Apgar score was to detect the effects of anesthesia on babies. Soon, it became adopted as a way of identifying which babies needed additional medical attention, such as more evaluation and intervention.

Full-term healthy babies receive Apgar scores of 7 to10. A score of 10 is rather rare so—all you parents who are perfectionists, please do not be disappointed! There is always a big difference between the temperatures in the mother's womb and in the delivery room. This temperature difference usually results in the baby having peripheral cyanosis (bluish hands and feet) and getting only one point for skin color. Thus, a total Apgar score may be 9 in an otherwise perfect baby.

In my opinion, the Apgar score is not as useful in premature babies as in term newborns. Tiny babies have naturally decreased muscle tone and most of them have breathing problems. Therefore, they almost always have lower scores.

A low Apgar score in the first few minutes of life does not predict poor long-term developmental outcomes, especially if it improves rapidly by 5 to 10 minutes of life, with proper interventions. However, low Apgar scores and the need for resuscitation beyond 10 to 15 minutes of life may be associated with poor neurological development in the future.

Taking measurements (weight, height, and head circumference)

One of the very first questions that are asked of the medical team is "How much does my baby weigh?" As a result, the baby's weight is checked relatively soon after birth and given to parents and family in pounds and kilograms, if desired. Doctors may also mention whether the baby's weight is within normal limits for their gestational age.

Sometimes, weight is more than what would be expected, based on known gestational age, and this is called "large for gestational age"—in short, "LGA." LGA babies may be born to mothers with various metabolic problems such as abnormal glucose control or diabetes.

Conversely, SGA means "small for gestational age." The most common reasons for this are smoking cigarettes during pregnancy, maternal high blood pressure, serious medical problems in the mother or congenital genetic problems, and infections of the fetus. It is always good to have a discussion with your doctor about why your baby is LGA or SGA if they are affected.

Soon after birth, we take the baby's vital signs (temperature, respiratory rate, and heart rate). The *normal respiratory rate* for a newborn baby falls between 40 and 60 breaths per minute. It should be noted that this is much higher than in the adult population. An increased respiratory rate may be a sign of problems with the lungs or heart, or caused by severe anemia. A lower respiratory rate can occur because of the effects of maternal medications, such as anesthesia, or some neurological problems and infections affecting the baby.

The *normal heart rate* for a newborn is usually 120 to 160 beats per minute. Heart rates that are higher or lower than average may be a result of various conditions originating in the heart, central nervous system, or other organs in the body.

The *normal axillary temperature* in a newborn is usually between 97.7 and 99.5F. A higher temperature in a baby right after birth may reflect maternal fever. A low body temperature may be the result of setting the environmental temperature in the delivery or operating room too low. Premature babies often present with low body temperature because of a lack of body fat and reduced ability to adjust their energy production. Both low and high body temperatures in a newborn baby may be indicative of infections or metabolic disorders. Small and premature babies are routinely placed on radiant warmer beds or in isolettes to prevent expected hypothermia (i.e. low body temperature).

Prophylactic measures that we perform right after birth

"Prophylaxis" is a term describing a procedure during which we try to prevent something from occurring. Usually, it requires some significant effort or resources. Therefore, it must be a worthwhile cause before deciding to do it on a full scale.

For newborn babies, there are specific prophylactic procedures that have been instituted and mandated by many states to prevent various medical conditions. When judging whether to establish a particular form of prevention, doctors consider whether a procedure can cause any harm or risk. Then they consider the possible benefits for all babies and society.

The following are the four most common prophylactic measures done to newborn babies after birth.

1. *Eye prophylaxis:* This is conducted to prevent gonococcal infection of the eyes, which may lead to blindness. It

is easy, safe, and ideally should be done within the first hour after birth. Most hospitals will use 0.5% antibiotic Erythromycin eye ointment for this purpose. In some areas, Tetracycline ointment or Silver Nitrate solution will be used instead. Erythromycin application is usually a well-tolerated procedure. The most common side effect of the eye prophylaxis is chemical irritation. This may occur 24 hours after the antibiotic application but will disappear 48 hours later.

2. *Vitamin K:* A vitamin K intramuscular injection is given to all newborns in the USA as a one-time injection to prevent severe bleeding caused by vitamin K deficiency. This dangerous bleeding is also known as "hemorrhagic disease of the newborn." Babies with this condition may develop severe bleeding in their brain, sometimes resulting in death. Some parents refuse vitamin K prophylaxis altogether, or they want to use an oral form instead, because of some concerns about a possible association between injectable vitamin K and cancer. The American Academy of Pediatrics concluded that the intramuscular form of vitamin K was superior to the oral form. After analyzing current available studies, they did not find evidence of any association between vitamin K and cancer. I have no doubt about this issue. A long time ago, I witnessed a two-week-old baby dying from hemorrhagic disease. That is enough for me to recommend the prophylaxis strongly unless risks of vitamin K are proven beyond any doubt.

3. *Hepatitis B vaccine:* Hepatitis B is a viral infection that can cause liver damage, or liver cancer, and ultimately may lead to death. Hepatitis B vaccine may protect you from contracting the disease. Typically, you contract Hepatitis B through contact with the blood or body fluids of an infected person. Most people who receive all three doses of the Hepatitis B vaccine will be well protected. In the USA, the first dose of the vaccine is being administered

to newborn babies before they are discharged home. We administer this vaccine intramuscularly into the muscle of buttocks or thighs. Most babies tolerate the vaccine very well. The most common problem afterwards is some swelling and soreness in the area of injection. Other side effects or serious issues are infrequent.

4. *Umbilical cord care*: The umbilical cord is clamped and cut within minutes after delivery but practices regarding the care of the umbilical cord vary. Some people leave it to dry on its own. In some nurseries, different agents such as triple dye, alcohol, silver sulfadiazine, and chlorohexidine are applied to it. The purpose of these agents is to prevent or reduce bacterial colonization and possibly reduce the risk of infection for babies. If a baby is tiny or requires immediate treatment, we may place catheters into the vessels located within the umbilical cord. These catheters can then be used to provide intravenous (IV) fluids and medications, and to draw blood for testing.

Three standard blood tests that doctors may order for newborn babies after birth

1. *Glucose levels*: Some babies are at higher risk of having low blood glucose levels after birth and need to be monitored for that eventuality. Glucose is a type of sugar that is necessary for the proper function of the brain. In situations when the glucose level is too low, a baby may stop breathing, have seizures, or present with temperature instability, poor feeding, or jitteriness. All premature babies, without exception, are at risk for low glucose levels. Other risk factors for low glucose levels in a baby include LGA, SGA, high red cell counts, and maternal diabetes. Whenever a low blood glucose level is discovered, nurses or doctors will try to feed the baby or give IV fluids to increase the level. Checking blood glucose levels is easy: it involves pricking the baby's heel and collecting

one drop of blood on a paper strip. Insertion of that strip into a portable machine gives results almost immediately.

2. *Checking a baby's blood type and the Coombs or DAT test*: There are many blood group systems, but two are of the most concern for pediatricians: the ABO system and the Rh system. In cases where a mother is "O type" in the ABO system or "Rh-negative" in the Rh system, it is recommended to check the baby's blood type. At the same time, we would also screen the baby for antibodies of maternal origin and whether these antibodies react with the baby's red blood cells. This last test is called an *"antibody screening test"* or a *"Coombs test."* Knowing the baby's blood type and the Coombs test result helps us assess the risk of them developing significant jaundice or anemia. This assessment will influence our decisions regarding further follow-up and treatment of jaundice if needed.

3. *Bilirubin levels*: Jaundice is a condition in which the skin of a newborn baby turns yellow, and it is due to an increased level of a chemical called "bilirubin." Most premature babies will have some jaundice. Many of them will need treatment with phototherapy because untreated very high bilirubin levels may lead to severe neurological problems. Nowadays, almost all nurseries screen babies for jaundice either by measuring the transcutaneous bilirubin level through the skin without any needle sticks or by checking the bilirubin level in the blood. Depending on the baby's age at the time of the test and the bilirubin level, the doctors will decide whether there is a need for treatment or additional follow-up tests.

Blood tests that are done in newborns when we suspect an infection

A newborn baby may require testing for infection in several situations. The first one would be when a mother has specific risk factors that increase the baby's chances of acquiring the infection.

Examples of these situations are if the mother has already developed an infection and is clinically ill, or if she carries bacteria in her body (GBS colonization) that does not cause disease in her but is potentially harmful to the baby.

When we talk about babies, almost any type of abnormal behavior or finding may be an early sign of infection. Problems such as irregular breathing, need for oxygen therapy, temperature instability, glucose problems, or poor feeding may prompt us to evaluate a baby for infection.

There are three standard tests that we may order if we suspect infection in a baby. Two of them, CBC (complete blood counts) and CRP (C-reactive protein), are indirect tests. They do not give you an absolute answer. If they are abnormal, they only raise your level of suspicion of infection. On the other hand, the third test—blood culture—is the most important. If the blood culture is positive, it always means that the baby has a bacterial infection in its body, and such a baby needs urgent treatment and further evaluation. Importantly, babies may also be infected by yeasts and viruses. However, the latter two are more challenging to diagnose on routine culture tests.

Screening

The newborn state screen and metabolic state screen

The newborn state screen is a screening test performed on all newborn babies in the USA and almost everywhere else. It's a test that may reveal whether your baby has a severe metabolic, genetic, or hematologic disease. Various states test for a different number of diseases. In olden days, we tested for only 4 to 5 disorders. Nowadays, with new laboratory techniques, states test for 50 or more conditions that otherwise would have been undetected for a long time until a child became symptomatic later in life.

Examples of the diseases that we screen for in the newborn state screen are:

- phenylketonuria;
- galactosemia;
- hypothyroidism;
- congenital adrenal hyperplasia;
- hemoglobinopathies; and
- organic academies.

The idea behind newborn state screening is that many of the disorders tested for can be modified and treated successfully if detected early. The screen is performed by taking a few drops of blood from the baby's heel and placing them on special laboratory paper. These samples are sent to the state lab and results are given to the birth hospital or your baby's pediatrician. As a parent, you should always ask and confirm with your pediatrician that your baby's newborn state screening is normal. Typically, this screening is performed within the first 48 hours of life, and in premature babies it is later repeated, often several times more.

Screening for cyanotic congenital heart disease using a pulse oximeter

All babies before discharge home undergo pulse oximetry screening. This test is performed using two sensors: one on the right hand and the other on a foot. If the readings are abnormal, one should suspect congenital heart disease and immediately conduct a more specific evaluation to confirm or rule out that diagnosis. Abnormal screening for congenital heart disease is urgent and always requires consultation with a neonatologist or pediatric cardiologist.

Hearing screening

In the USA, we screen all newborn babies for hearing deficits before they go home. Premature babies are at higher risk of developing hearing deficits than term newborns. The test is performed by placing leads on the baby's head and connecting those leads to a machine. The testing machine can read brain waves created in response to sounds and assess if the baby has a hearing deficit. The test serves only as a screening so, if a baby fails the test, we refer them for a repeat hearing test within a month or for more formal evaluation by an audiologist or an ear, nose and throat specialist.

CHAPTER 7

Kangaroo Care

O ften, parents ask me how they can help their premature baby who is staying in the neonatal intensive care unit (NICU). My answer is always the same. There are two things they can do for their little one: provide breast milk and do "Kangaroo Care" (KC).

In this chapter, I will talk about KC. It has many benefits and there are few dangers. I will list and explain the most important of both.

Basic information

KC resembles what kangaroos do to their babies after birth. Kangaroo mothers have a physiological pocket on the belly where they put their babies to carry them around.

In a NICU, **KC** involves placing a newborn baby, dressed only in a diaper and head cap, on the bare chest of the mother or father. Then, we cover the baby with blankets to protect them from drafts and ensure stable body temperature. If the baby tolerates it well, parents can hold their baby for several hours.

While the baby is receiving KC, a nurse will be monitoring their condition, paying particular attention to body temperature and breathing pattern.

I want to emphasize that babies receiving KC will always remain on their monitors and ventilators, and continue receiving all necessary treatments.

What is the lowest weight or gestational age of a baby who can receive KC? There is no such thing as a minimum gestational age or weight for this care. More important is whether the baby is stable enough. Often, premature babies have more stable vital signs parameters in their mother's arms than when placed alone in an incubator.

Benefits of Kangaroo Care

Doctors and nurses describe numerous benefits from KC, and both parents and the baby can benefit from it.

Benefits for the baby

KC improves weight gain over time and facilitates an earlier discharge home: Without a doubt, close bonding between a mother and her baby positively influences her breast milk supply. Breast milk is like GOLD for extremely premature babies. One of the most desirable outcomes expected of premature babies is consistent and proper weight gain. The best tool to achieve this result is having maternal breast milk available for each baby. Babies fed breast milk will tolerate feedings better and will likely receive many other health benefits from it.

KC helps with body temperature regulation: Very premature babies are at risk of developing low body temperature. This is due to many factors: less body fat, a larger body surface area, inadequate amount of energy resources, and reduced brain ability to preserve thermoregulation. Surprisingly, we often observe that babies placed on their mothers' chests and covered with blankets rarely have any temperature problems.

More sleep time and better quality of sleep: It is unfortunate, but a NICU is a very noisy environment and probably not the best place for babies to sleep. Well, we do not give them a choice if they are born prematurely and need our care. Several studies found that infants who were receiving regular KC had more sleep time, and their brains matured faster, achieving greater complexity.

Decreased mortality and shorter hospitalization time: KC for premature babies and babies born with low birth weight should be promoted, particularly in low-resource countries. In places where adequate neonatal care is not available, where doctors do not have incubators or intravenous (IV) fluids, KC can be life-saving. Cochrane reviewers looked at many clinical studies and provided a summary of the findings. "Kangaroo Mother Care" was associated with decreased mortality rates, reduced rates of infections, and faster discharge home.

Benefits for the mother and father

KC promotes bonding and decreases stress: The hardest part of having your baby in a NICU is being separated from it. Although some NICUs have private rooms where parents can stay with their babies all the time, this is not a common practice. Even when a hospital has adequate infrastructure, parents often have other children and obligations and cannot stay with the baby for a prolonged time. Providing KC allows for closer bonding with the baby and has the power to decrease parental stress levels.

KC helps you to produce more breast milk: Skin-to-skin care with your baby is the best tool in facilitating breast milk production. It has been established in many earlier studies that breast milk is the best medicine for premature babies, particularly micro-preemies. Premature delivery and separation of the mother from her baby have a negative impact on maternal milk production. KC is a great way to rectify some of those problems. Close bonding between mother and baby always positively influences maternal milk production.

KC improves your confidence that you can take care of your baby: Often, after the birth of extremely premature babies or micro-preemies, parents are afraid to touch them. They do not know how to care for their baby, how to take their temperature, how to change a diaper, and so on. Providing KC allows them to observe their baby closely and often increases their confidence. They are quickly convinced that the whole experience is not that scary, and that they are ready for more challenges than "just" holding their baby.

Potential risks of Kangaroo Care

KC may have some risks. The obvious ones are that your tiny baby may not tolerate it well and may have temperature instability or breathing problems. The bedside nurse will monitor your baby for any signs of intolerance and intervene if necessary. Another danger is that KC requires placement of your baby in a prone position. Positioning a baby on their belly is generally discouraged in full-term babies to prevent sudden infant death syndrome. We are not aware of any increased risk for severe apneas in preterm babies receiving KC. However, babies receiving KC in the NICU must be continuously monitored.

CHAPTER 8

Respiratory distress syndrome

Respiratory distress syndrome (RDS) is a lung disease occurring mostly in premature babies due to lung immaturity and surfactant deficiency.

RDS is a diagnosis given to babies with respiratory symptoms because of their anatomical and chemical immaturity (the latter is due to surfactant deficiency in the lungs). Most newborns with RDS are premature babies. Some early-term babies and full-term newborns may also be affected but this is rare. Among premature and full-term babies, newborns delivered by mothers who had diabetes during pregnancy have a higher risk of developing RDS.

The lungs of fetuses undergo the maturation process in utero. That involves growing a number of bronchial tree branches and increasing the production of a chemical called "surfactant." An increase in the number of airways and alveoli (tiny air bubbles in the lungs where oxygen—CO_2 gas exchange occurs) contributes to increasing the surface area of gas exchange in our lungs. That process continues until birth and beyond.

Surfactant is a complex chemical substance that covers alveoli. Its role is to prevent alveoli from collapsing. In other words, it is necessary for our lungs to function properly.

When a baby does not have enough airways and the surfactant is reduced, or malfunctioning, the baby will develop RDS. The condition may also be due to genetic defects. However, only a minority of babies with RDS have a genetic condition affecting the production of surfactant. Sadly, RDS caused by genetic mutations usually has a very severe clinical course.

If you have read older articles or books on this subject, doctors may have used different terms to describe RDS. In the past, it used to be also called "hyaline membrane disease" or "premature lung disease."

How common is respiratory distress syndrome in premature babies?

The strongest risk factors for RDS are low gestational age at birth and low birth weight. Additional risk factors are maternal diabetes and hypoxia (low oxygen levels in the fetus before delivery). RDS is also more frequent among male babies.

RDS is seen in 95% to 98% of babies born at 22 to 24 weeks of gestation, and 25% to 50% of babies born at 28 to 32 weeks of gestational age will have the condition. Its incidence drops to 5% at 34 weeks of gestational age and to 1% at 37 weeks. Although it is uncommon for babies born at more than 37 weeks to have RDS, it is not impossible.

Can respiratory distress syndrome be prevented?

There are two ways to prevent or modify the course of RDS.

1. Preventing premature birth, or at least delaying it, is the best way to decrease the incidence and severity of RDS.
2. Having regular prenatal care, proper nutrition, and good life habits all contribute to a healthier fetus and pregnancy.

Also, there are some medications (called "tocolytics") that can be given to slow down premature contractions and labor progression.

If a mother is already in premature labor or threatened early labor, the administration of steroids (Betamethasone) to her can significantly increase the maturity of fetal lungs and decrease the incidence and severity of RDS in a premature baby.

There are several positive outcomes for a baby if at least 24 to 48 hours pass between administration of maternal steroids and delivery of the baby:

- A decrease in neonatal mortality.
- Decreased incidence and severity of RDS after birth.
- A reduction in the rate of intraventricular hemorrhage (bleeding in the brain).

Steroids may affect maternal blood pressure and glucose levels. However, more severe side effects are rare. Concerns about the possibility of an increase in infections in mothers or their babies have been unfounded.

Effects of repeated courses of steroids on premature babies' long-term outcomes are still debated. Therefore, doctors are cautious before offering second or third rounds of steroids to a mother who returns 2 or 3 weeks later—again in premature labor because she has not delivered yet.

What are the symptoms of respiratory distress syndrome in preemies?

Symptoms in babies with RDS are non-specific. This means that the same symptoms can occur in other respiratory diseases that newborns may have.

The following are symptoms in newborn babies with breathing problems:

- Increased respiratory rate (also called "tachypnea").
- Grunting (an expiratory noise while a baby is breathing).

- Nasal flaring (movements of sides of the nose while a baby is breathing).
- Retractions (sinking movements of the chest wall below the lower ribs when a baby is inhaling air).
- Decreased breath sounds when doctors listen to the lungs.
- Reduced levels of oxygen and increased levels of carbon dioxide in blood gas tests.
- Decreased levels of hemoglobin oxygen saturation (visible on the bedside monitor: normal values are considered to be above 92%).

If a baby has increased respiratory rate and also presents with nasal flaring, grunting, and retractions, we often say that they have "increased work of breathing."

How is the diagnosis of respiratory distress syndrome made?

Diagnosis of RDS in a newborn baby is always presumptive. There is no single test that could confirm this diagnosis with 100% certainty at the bedside. Whenever we have a premature baby or a baby with additional risks for RDS, and respiratory symptoms are present, we presume that the baby has RDS. A chest x-ray may be helpful, but it is not diagnostic because other conditions (like Group B Streptococcus pneumonia) can mimic RDS on a chest x-ray. The clinical course consistent with RDS is of a disease that shows symptoms developing soon after birth: increased work of breathing and need for extra oxygen. Respiratory symptoms will be gradually getting worse if not treated.

How do we evaluate the severity of respiratory distress syndrome in babies?

Evaluation of the severity of RDS relies on clinical observation, physical examination, chest x-ray, and blood gases.

While conducting an examination, we pay particular attention to the amount of oxygen needed by the baby and the amount of work of breathing: severity of retractions and respiratory rate. Need for additional oxygen over 50%, deep subcostal chest retractions, and a high respiratory rate of more than 100 breaths per minute usually signify severe RDS.

On chest x-ray, severe RDS is defined by reduced lung expansion and poor aeration of the lung fields. If the doctor describes the lungs as entirely whited-out, that probably means severe RDS.

Blood gases allow us to assess the efficiency of gas exchange taking place in the lungs and the chemical–metabolic balance in the body. Low oxygen levels, high carbon dioxide levels, and acidosis mean more severe RDS in a baby.

Treatment of respiratory distress syndrome

The treatment of RDS is mostly symptomatic and, with the one exception described below, it is non-specific. We want to support a baby with different measures to maintain the body's physiologic functions without disturbing the baby too much. That way, we allow natural recovery processes to take place, and we promote self-healing of the lungs.

After birth, the baby's lungs accelerate the maturation process. Eventually, the lungs reach the level where the baby will be breathing more comfortably and will not need supplementary oxygen any more.

Depending on the severity of RDS, we can use one or several of the treatments described below:

1. *NPO (a Latin abbreviation for "nothing by mouth"*: Babies with fast respiratory rates are not allowed to breastfeed or bottle-feed because of the risk of aspiration. It is difficult for them to coordinate breathing, sucking, and swallowing when their respiratory rate is above 60 to 70 breaths per minute. Whenever a baby's respiratory rate is above

those levels, we have two choices: give milk via a plastic tube directly into the stomach or stop feedings and start intravenous fluids.

2. _Antibiotics:_ Most babies with moderate or severe respiratory problems will be treated with antibiotics. After birth, we never know for sure whether there is an ongoing infection. We do not want to take the risk of leaving a potential infection untreated. We prefer to evaluate for infection and start each baby with RDS on antibiotics. If a baby gets better and our evaluation is negative, in most cases, we will stop antibiotics 48 hours later.

3. _Oxygen_: Many babies with RDS have decreased oxygen levels in their bodies due to their lower ability to absorb oxygen from their immature lungs. As a result, they require an increased concentration of oxygen for breathing. Extra oxygen can be provided to them in different ways. If they do not have increased work of breathing, we can provide additional oxygen via the plastic box surrounding their head called an "Oxyhood." If a baby has increased work of breathing, we can add supplementary oxygen into the circuit of a nasal cannula, a continuous positive airway pressure (CPAP) device, or a ventilator (see below for explanations).

4. _Supporting respiratory efforts in a baby_: If a baby has significantly increased work of breathing as described above, we have to support its efforts using one of the three following devices:

A: **Nasal cannula:** This is a small, flexible, plastic tube inserted in a baby's nose that provides a flow of air with additional oxygen. Nasal cannulas are used in milder cases of RDS.

B: **CPAP device:** This is a device that offers extra pressure for the baby during the expiratory phase of its breathing efforts. Air with oxygen flows to the baby through special cannulas inserted in the nose or through the small mask placed around the baby's nose. This type of respiratory support is used in babies with moderately increased work of breathing.

C: **A ventilator "breathing machine"**: Babies who have a severe form of RDS with abnormal levels of oxygen and carbon dioxide in their blood need a ventilator. A ventilator is a machine that provides external artificial breaths for the baby through the plastic tube placed in the baby's trachea (windpipe). If needed, supplementary oxygen is provided into the respiratory circuit as well. It is difficult to predict how long a newborn baby will need a ventilator. Most babies born at 28 to 32 weeks will require mechanical ventilation for no more than a few days. Babies born at fewer than 28 weeks may need a ventilator for a week, a month, or even several months. The duration of mechanical ventilation will depend on the gestational age, birth weight, and on other accompanying conditions and complications that the baby may develop during their neonatal intensive care unit (NICU) stay.

5. *Blood transfusion*: If a baby is severely anemic.

6. *Blood pressure support with medications*: If a baby is hypotensive (hypotension = low blood pressure).

7. *Surfactant administration*: Surfactant is the only medication that is specific to the treatment of RDS. It was introduced into our treatment repertoire in early1990, and now I can say that it is an essential medication in neonatology. Surfactant is a complex substance that contains phospholipids and unique types of proteins. It can be produced synthetically or obtained from natural preparations of extracts from calf lung lavage, minced bovine, or porcine lungs. The latter, natural forms of surfactant, are more popular, better understood, and known to us—and probably more effective in treating RDS. Surfactant is a liquid medication that needs to be administered directly into a baby's lungs. At this time, it can only be done by inserting a catheter or breathing

tube (an endotracheal tube) into the baby's trachea and injecting the surfactant down into the lungs. In the future, we might be able to provide surfactant by nebulization in aerosolized form, but this method is still under development and in research trials.

Outcomes and prognosis of RDS in premature babies

In most cases, RDS will improve after several days and the baby will slowly grow out of the condition.

In micro-preemies and extremely premature babies, RDS may evolve into chronic lung disease, also known as "bronchopulmonary dysplasia" (see Chapter 11). In the acute phase, a small group of babies may develop a complication called "air leak" or "pneumothorax." In pneumothorax, a tiny portion of lung ruptures and air leaks out from the lung into the space between the internal chest wall and the lung. That, in turn, causes the lungs' compression and prevents them from expanding and functioning correctly. Pneumothorax always develops suddenly and can be dangerous. It usually leads to acute deterioration of the clinical condition. The good news is that, if recognized quickly, pneumothorax is treatable. After prompt treatment, a baby can still completely recover from pneumothorax and RDS.

Questions to ask if your baby is being treated for respiratory distress syndrome

1. How much supplementary oxygen does my baby need for breathing?
2. How severe is RDS in my baby?
3. Does my baby need surfactant and a ventilator to treat their RDS?
4. Is your hospital adequately equipped and experienced to treat RDS in my baby? (In most cases where a baby needs surfactant and a ventilator, they should be treated in a NICU level 3 or 4).

In summary

RDS is a pulmonary condition occurring mostly in premature babies due to lung immaturity and surfactant deficiency. Treatment of RDS is primarily non-specific and supportive. Surfactant is the medication that can be administered to patients with moderate and severe RDS, especially if those babies are on a ventilator.

CHAPTER 9

Apnea of prematurity—my baby periodically stops breathing

I t is always scary for parents to hear that their baby is stopping breathing for short periods of time.

Apnea of prematurity is defined as a cessation of breathing in a premature baby for 15 to 20 seconds, or a shorter duration if it is associated with low oxygen levels and a low heart rate. Before making a diagnosis of apnea of prematurity, other causes of apnea should be considered and ruled out.

Apnea is a common condition in premature babies. Fifty percent of babies born between 33 and 35 weeks of gestational age develop it. Most babies born before 28 weeks will suffer from apnea that will need treatment. Often, persistent apnea will be the only reason why a baby still needs to be hospitalized in a NICU, leading to frustration among family members who want to have their baby discharged home as soon as possible.

Unfortunately, in many micro-preemies and extremely premature babies, resolution of apnea may be reached only after 43 to 44 weeks of corrected gestational age (3 to 4 weeks after the pregnancy's expected due date).

Why do premature babies develop apnea?

Apnea of prematurity is caused by the physiological immaturity of the respiratory center in the brain and the anatomical immaturity of the upper airways. In healthy people, the brain respiratory center provides a constant respiratory drive. This regulatory mechanism can adapt to quickly changing levels of oxygen and carbon dioxide in mature babies, slowing or increasing respiratory rate whenever needed. In premature babies, the regulatory process may malfunction, leading to so-called "central apnea." In other words, central apnea occurs when the brain provides inadequate stimulation to the muscles responsible for breathing movements.

Patency of the upper airways is also crucial for air movement during breathing efforts. Many premature babies develop "obstructive apnea" (blockage in the airways) due to their narrow airways and weak muscles surrounding those airways.

In most situations, premature babies have so-called "mixed apnea," meaning that both factors (lack of central stimulation and obstruction of the airways) play a role.

What are the symptoms of apnea of prematurity?

As said above, apnea is defined as a cessation of breathing for 15 to 20 seconds, or less if it is accompanied by low oxygen levels or a low heart rate. Every premature baby who stays in a NICU is monitored using cardiorespiratory and pulse oximeter monitors. The cardiorespiratory monitor allows us to watch and record the baby's respiratory rate and heart rate. The pulse oximeter measures hemoglobin saturation, which is an indicator of oxygen levels in the baby's blood. Even if a nurse is not present at the baby's bedside all the time, monitors will ring alarms whenever the baby's vital parameters fall outside of the normal range.

Detecting pauses in breathing effort is relatively easy by watching a baby or reviewing recordings from the monitors. However, determining that apneic episodes are due to prematurity requires going through other possible differential diagnoses to rule them out.

Is it apnea of prematurity, or could it be something else?

Whenever a baby presents to us with apnea, before making the diagnosis of apnea of prematurity, we should consider other options. We need to go over the list of conditions for which apnea may also be a symptom. Let's look at some of these differential diagnoses below.

Sepsis—generalized infection

If a previously stable baby develops apnea later than one week after birth, one should consider infection as a cause. Extremely premature babies and micro-preemies are very prone to infections. Their immune system is undeveloped. They did not receive enough antibodies from their mothers due to the shortened pregnancy, and many are exposed to central lines and ventilators that carry an increased risk of catching an infection.

Babies affected by infection may have symptoms other than apnea: low body temperature, exacerbated breathing problems, low blood pressure, low or high sugar levels, and feeding intolerance.

To rule out infection, doctors will order various tests but, at minimum, complete blood counts and blood cultures (we may also test spinal fluid and urine for infections). If a baby has symptoms that could be caused by infection, we often start antibiotics before the diagnosis of sepsis is confirmed.

Anemia

Premature babies often have low levels of red blood cells. Red blood cells carry oxygen to our organs and tissues. Therefore, it is crucial to have an adequate amount of them. Premature babies may be born with a low number of red blood cells, or they may develop anemia after birth due to frequent blood draws and their bone marrow not being able to produce red blood cells quickly enough. We know that severe anemia may exacerbate already existing apnea of prematurity or cause apneic events by itself. Most clinicians would consider blood transfusion in a baby with apnea and significant anemia with a hematocrit of less than 25%. Hematocrit measures the proportion of red blood cells in the blood, and results are reported in percentages. Adults have hematocrit levels around 42%, and full-term babies around 55%.

Necrotic enterocolitis

Necrotic enterocolitis is a severe inflammatory and infectious disease of bowel loops, occurring more often in babies born at fewer than 28 weeks of gestational age. Apnea may be one of the presenting symptoms. However, almost always, babies will also have severe feeding intolerance with gastric residuals, abdominal distension, and bloody stools. Necrotic enterocolitis is treated with antibiotics, intravenous (IV) fluids, and sometimes with surgery.

Intraventricular hemorrhage

Intraventricular hemorrhage (IVH) occurs in very premature babies. The rupture of small blood vessels in the brain is a cause. Blood enters the ventricles and may compress on vital areas of the brain. In some patients, IVH may evolve into hydrocephalus. When a baby is developing IVH or, later, when a baby suffers from hydrocephalus, they may present with significant apneic episodes. Brain imaging with a head ultrasound or a head CAT scan will confirm or rule out the diagnosis of IVH.

Seizure disorder

Some newborn babies may develop seizures in infancy. In some cases, apneic episodes may be the first or only sign of seizures. To confirm or rule out seizure disorder, doctors will order an electric study of the brain called an "EEG."

Hypoglycemia

Hypoglycemia is a medical term used to describe abnormally low sugar levels (glucose) in the body. It may be accompanied by apnea if these glucose levels are very low. Hypoglycemia is more common in babies born very small or very large for their gestational age (SGA or LGA) and in babies of diabetic mothers.

Neonatal encephalopathy (due to low oxygen levels at and around birth time)

Prolonged exposure of the baby to low oxygen levels during labor and delivery may lead to brain damage called "neonatal encephalopathy." Apnea may be one of the symptoms of this condition. It is important to emphasize that neonatal encephalopathy occurs in both preterm and term babies. We will suspect neonatal encephalopathy when babies have a history of heart decelerations during labor and were given a very low Apgar score at birth.

Congenital anomalies of the airways

Various developmental anomalies that affect the patency of the airways may be the cause of apnea. Sometimes airway anomalies are evident during an external examination. However, often an ear, nose, and throat (ENT) specialist is needed to conduct a thorough examination of the upper and lower airways in a baby to rule out this diagnosis conclusively. Symptoms such as noisy breathing or choking episodes while feeding are suggestive of problems with the airways and may require an ENT consult.

Feeding problems in a premature baby

Oral feeding is a complex task for a baby. It involves three separate actions that need to be well coordinated: sucking, swallowing, and breathing. Many premature babies born below 34 weeks of gestational age do not know how to eat by mouth and have to learn that skill. During the learning process, they may have apneic episodes during feedings or right after. Also, many premature babies suffer from gastroesophageal reflux due to a physiologically weak esophageal sphincter muscle. As a result, stomach contents can travel back up into the esophagus, mouth, or nose. Severe esophageal reflux may result in aspiration of stomach contents into the lungs.

Doctors still debate how much reflux contributes to apnea in premature babies, and whether reflux treatment helps at all. However, it is plausible that severe reflux may be contributing to the severity of apnea in premature babies. Whether to treat it is another big question.

Treatment of mothers in labor with opiates and magnesium sulfate

Opioid medications are used for control of labor pains. Opiates easily cross the placenta and enter the baby's circulation before birth. It is well known that maternal opioids can cause respiratory depression and apnea in babies during the first few hours after birth.

Magnesium sulfate is used in mothers to control blood pressure or slow down premature labor contractions. It causes muscle weakness and sleepiness in babies and may also lead to apnea after birth.

Whenever apnea in a baby is due to maternal medications, it manifests itself soon after birth and it gets better quickly. It usually resolves within 24 to 48 hours after delivery once the baby excretes all the medicines out of their system.

How do we treat apnea of prematurity?

Not all apneas of prematurity require treatment. Clinicians will start treating apnea of prematurity when at least one of the following conditions is met:

1. Apneic <u>episodes are persistent</u>, prolonged, and accompanied by oxygen saturation below 85%.
2. The baby requires <u>frequent vigorous stimulation</u> or artificial ventilation before restarting its breathing efforts.

Once therapy for apnea is started, it is usually needed until 34 weeks of corrected gestational age. In micro-preemies, it is not unusual to continue it until 44 weeks. Doctors treat apnea of prematurity by providing appropriate respiratory support and with a medicine called "caffeine." Depending on the severity of the premature baby's lung disease and apnea, various types of respiratory support may be needed:

*   A nasal cannula.
*   A continuous positive airway pressure (CPAP) device.
*   A ventilator.

Each technique is capable of providing a mixture of air with additional oxygen as needed for the baby. I describe these three respiratory techniques in <u>Chapters 8 and 11</u>.

Caffeine is a chemical substance also found in coffee and tea. We can give it to a baby orally or intravenously. It keeps us awake, but it also stimulates a baby's respirations. It has been known about for a long time and is well tolerated by babies. The two most commonly occurring side effects are increased heart rate (tachycardia) and gastroesophageal reflux. If doctors are concerned about caffeine toxicity, they can measure caffeine levels in the blood and its dose can be easily adjusted.

In extremely premature babies and micro-preemies, caffeine is used prophylactically to facilitate the discontinuation of mechanical ventilation or to avoid it altogether.

What is the prognosis in apnea of prematurity?

All premature babies outgrow apnea of prematurity with time. For some, it happens around 34 to 35 weeks of gestational age but, in the tiniest babies, apnea may persist until 44 weeks of postconceptional age. If apnea of prematurity does not get better or resolve over time, apneic episodes are likely to be due to causes other than just prematurity.

CHAPTER 10

Yellow skin— newborn jaundice or hyperbilirubinemia

J aundice in a newborn is the most common condition neo-natologists encounter after birth in both preterm and term babies. Jaundice is a term used to describe the presence of yellow skin color in a baby. It is caused by skin deposition of *bilirubin*, a naturally occurring chemical in our body. Hence, among medics, this condition is also called "hyperbilirubin-emia." Bilirubin levels in our body depend on its production, elimination, and reabsorption. Bilirubin is produced during the breakdown of red blood cells, and it circulates around the body. Some of it enters the liver, where it undergoes transformation called "conjugation," allowing it to be excreted into the bowel loops with bile and then excreted with the stool. During passage through the gut, some of the bilirubin gets reabsorbed into the circulation again.

If I simplify, I can divide all types of jaundice into two groups: indirect hyperbilirubinemia (non-obstructive jaundice) and direct hyperbilirubinemia (cholestatic jaundice). Both chemical compounds, "indirect" and "direct," can be measured in the blood. First, I will focus on the more popular form: non-obstructive jaundice disease, which affects most premature babies. In Part 2, I will explain cholestatic jaundice.

Part 1: Jaundice due to indirect hyperbilirubinemia = non-obstructive jaundice

Three processes can influence and lead to significant jaundice in the newborn baby: decreased elimination of bilirubin, increased production, and increased reabsorption of bilirubin from the gut.

Jaundice due to decreased elimination of bilirubin

Disorders of elimination will contribute to a sustained and increasing bilirubin load in the circulation. All newborn babies, and particularly premature babies, have naturally deficient liver enzymes normally helping to eliminate bilirubin from our bodies. Additionally, some genetic and hormonal defects can impair liver enzymes further. Birth is a potent stimulus that enhances liver enzymes activity. Therefore, over 1 to 4 weeks after delivery, liver enzymes will reach levels allowing them to tackle normal loads of bilirubin and jaundice will resolve on its own. In the meantime, many babies will require treatment.

Jaundice due to increased production of bilirubin

In some situations, the production of bilirubin increases significantly. Examples of such conditions include blood group incompatibilities, enzymatic defects of red cells, structural abnormalities of red cells, bacterial and viral infections, and traumatic delivery. Blood group incompatibilities are quite common. However, the other conditions listed earlier are rare causes of jaundice. Blood incompatibility occurs when the mother is Rh-negative and the baby is Rh-positive, or when a mother is group "O" and the baby is either "A" or "B." When blood incompatibility exists, the mother passes specific antibodies to the baby and these antibodies facilitate destruction of the baby's red cells, thereby contributing to an increased bilirubin load.

Jaundice due to increased reabsorption of bilirubin from the gut

During the first week of life, premature babies eat very little and receive most of their nutrients intravenously, resulting in relative starvation, occasional dehydration, and delayed meconium passage (meconium = first bowel movement). This, in turn, will lead to increased reabsorption of bilirubin from the gut back into the circulation, thereby increasing the total bilirubin load in the body.

Is jaundice dangerous for newborn babies?

For the vast majority of babies, probably 99%, jaundice is a benign condition that resolves over time either on its own or with phototherapy. In cases where bilirubin rises rapidly to very high levels, the condition may be dangerous and lead to severe neurologic complications and even death.

What are the symptoms of jaundice?

The predominant symptom of newborn jaundice is yellowish skin color. Usually, you start seeing yellow skin color first on the face and in the white areas of the eyes (sclera). It later spreads in a downward direction covering chest, abdomen, and legs. In the olden days, doctors believed that they could assess the severity of jaundice based only on visual examination of the baby's skin color. However, data shows that visual estimations are notoriously inaccurate, and it would be dangerous to rely solely on visual inspection when assessing newborn jaundice—thus the need for blood tests. Babies who have jaundice due to blood type incompatibility and hemolysis may present with anemia, so pale skin may also be an accompanying finding.

Babies who have very high, or extremely high, bilirubin levels may have neurological symptoms such as lethargy, abnormal muscle tone, or even seizures. In rare situations, when a baby has jaundice due to an obstruction in the liver (see the later discussion of cholestatic jaundice), the baby may have greenish–yellowish skin color and their stools may be colorless or pale.

How do we diagnose and evaluate newborn jaundice?

Bilirubin levels

As I explained earlier, bilirubin is the chemical directly responsible for jaundice. We can measure the amount of bilirubin in a baby by using two different techniques: through the skin (transcutaneous) or a blood test. The transcutaneous method is non-invasive (no needle prick) and painless. It also provides results immediately. However, the disadvantage of this technique is that it measures only total bilirubin without differentiating between direct and indirect bilirubin, and it underestimates bilirubin values at higher levels. Additionally, it is less useful for tiny babies, and it cannot be reliably used after phototherapy has been started. Blood measurements of bilirubin levels are much more accurate and provide information on both direct and indirect bilirubin.

After we obtain bilirubin values, we plot them on nomograms (graphs developed after observing thousands of babies with jaundice) or bilirubin tables according to each baby's age and risk factors. These tools help us decide whether a patient needs treatment and future follow-up. It is essential to know that bilirubin levels always increase during the first 3 to 5 days, then reach a plateau and eventually decrease to typical adult values. In very small babies, the whole process may take several weeks.

Albumin levels

Albumin is a type of protein in the blood to which bilirubin tends to attach. Interestingly, bilirubin that is carried by albumins is less likely to cause brain damage. Therefore, the more albumin a baby has, the less likely they are to suffer neurological consequences from abnormally high bilirubin levels. Albumin is measured in a blood sample. It is a quick test that most hospitals can do. We do not measure albumin levels in every baby with jaundice—only in babies who have bilirubin at the levels close to the point where we would consider performing double volume exchange blood transfusion (see later).

Blood type in the baby and mother

All pregnant women have their blood type determined during pregnancy and, if it had not been done before, it would be done in a labor room. Doctors need to know the mother's blood type in case there is an emergency—for example, she has post-partum bleeding or needs emergency surgery. Also, knowing the mother's blood type allows us to determine whether the baby is at risk of having blood type incompatibility and, subsequently, a hemolytic reaction with jaundice.

Direct antiglobulin test (known as a "DAT test"; in the past, called a "Coombs test")

We do this direct antiglobulin blood test to find out whether there is a reaction between the maternal antibodies and the baby's red blood cells. It is needed when the mother and baby have incompatible blood types, as described earlier. The test proves that there is an ongoing hemolytic process in the baby's circulation, causing increased destruction of their red blood cells and leading to anemia and jaundice.

Complete blood count

A complete blood count (CBC) is a test looking at different types of cells in the blood. It is helpful in cases where there is blood type incompatibility between mother and baby, and there is a hemolytic process confirmed by a positive DAT test. The values we look at in CBC are numbers of red blood cells and the amount of hemoglobin. These two values will tell us whether the baby is anemic or not.

Blood smear

Obtaining a blood smear involves using a microscope to look at different cells in the blood and their shapes. Certain types of blood diseases in which red blood cells are misshaped can lead to hemolysis and increased bilirubin production. Examples of these blood disorders are spherocytosis or elliptocytosis (whereby red blood cells are in the shape of a sphere or an oval).

Measurements of enzymes such as G6PD or pyruvate kinase enzyme

Deficiencies of some enzymes may contribute to increased or prolonged jaundice. In rare cases where we do not have a precise diagnosis and cause of severe jaundice, we can measure these enzymes. We do not perform these tests in every situation.

Other tests

There will be rare situations where, after doing most or all the tests mentioned earlier, we will still not have a diagnosis regarding the cause of severe jaundice in a baby. Numerous very specialized tests are available to us, but they are beyond the scope of this chapter. We can test babies for congenital metabolic diseases, endocrine abnormalities, inherited defects, infections, and many other problems.

How do we treat newborn jaundice?

Not all cases of jaundice require treatment. However, probably 80% of babies born before 32 weeks will need at least phototherapy. The chosen therapy will depend on the severity and cause of the jaundice disease, but could include:

- phototherapy—the most important;
- nutrition and hydration;
- immunoglobulin infusions;
- double volume exchange blood transfusion;
- supplemental blood transfusion; or
- phenobarbital.

Phototherapy

Phototherapy with proper nutrition and hydration is the most important treatment modality for clinically significant jaundice. It uses narrow-spectrum lights and works by transforming bilirubin into soluble compounds that can be excreted from the baby's body. We provide phototherapy using banked overhead lamps, spotlights (one bulb), or biliblankets. A biliblanket looks literally like a flat blanket with tiny LED bulbs in it. It is flexible, so we can use it during feedings and different procedures. For phototherapy to be effective, we have to expose as much of the baby's skin as possible to it. Usually, the baby will be lying naked under phototherapy lamps wearing only a "bikini" diaper and protective eye goggles. If the baby requires only single phototherapy, we may lay them on the biliblanket, then put a shirt over them and swaddle them with a regular baby blanket. Double phototherapy is provided by lying the baby on the biliblanket or table lamps and then placing a second lamp over the baby's body.

In olden days, we had to be very careful not to overheat a baby with phototherapy. Nowadays, this complication occurs very rarely because modern lamps do not produce that much heat any more.

Are there any complications of phototherapy?

Phototherapy has been around for several decades and millions of newborn babies have received the treatment without any complications. In the past, before we had modern phototherapy lamps, babies could have suffered from overheating. However, nowadays, this occurs very rarely.

Babies who have obstructive jaundice or an increased amount of direct bilirubin (also called "conjugated bilirubin") may develop "bronze baby syndrome." This is greyish-brown discoloration of the skin and urine, but it is not life-threatening. Babies with congenital porphyria (a rare metabolic disorder) may react with severe purpura and a blistering bullous rash. If we notice such severe photosensitivity in any baby, we will stop phototherapy right away.

Some people are concerned about the effects of phototherapy on immature eyes. To prevent any eye damage, we cover babies' eyes with special goggles to eliminate any risks from prolonged exposure to intense light.

Nutrition and hydration

Nutrition and proper hydration are essential in managing jaundice. They help to ensure the uptake of bilirubin by the liver and kidneys, which participate in its excretion. Intestinal peristalsis and frequent stooling will also contribute to decreased reabsorption of bilirubin from bowel loops, thereby reducing the total bilirubin load in the body.

Immunoglobulin infusions

Immunoglobulin (IgG) infusions may play a role in hemolytic jaundice due to blood type incompatibilities (ABO or Rh). The exact mechanism of their effectiveness is unknown. We theorize that immunoglobulins may be able to block sites on a baby's red blood cells to which maternal antibodies would want to attach to cause their breakdown. Preventing the destruction of the baby's red blood cells will help to decrease the final bilirubin load, which is responsible for neonatal jaundice. Usually, babies tolerate IgG infusion very well, but sometimes rare side effects can occur. To decrease the likelihood of adverse reactions, we infuse immunoglobulins over several hours and closely monitor the baby's vital signs (temperature, respiratory rate, heart rate, and blood pressure).

Double volume exchange blood transfusion

When bilirubin is rising extremely fast, or it is at the level likely to cause neurological damage, exchange transfusion is indicated. For this procedure, we request blood from the blood bank that is compatible with the baby's blood and does not contain any antibodies against the baby's red blood cells. Typically, we perform the procedure using one or two centrally placed umbilical catheters (an umbilical catheter is a small sterile plastic tube inserted into the umbilicus and connected to a syringe, intravenous (IV) bag, or bag containing the blood). During the procedure, we remove small amounts of the baby's blood and replace it with the blood from the blood bank. The goal is to replace the double volume of the baby's blood, thereby achieving a significant decrease in bilirubin levels. Nowadays, we don't perform exchange transfusions very often. This is thanks to very effective phototherapy lamps and the availability of IgG for hemolytic jaundice.

Supplemental blood transfusion

Supplementary blood transfusion is not jaundice treatment per se, but it may be needed in hemolytic jaundice when the disease is also accompanied by anemia. Hyperbilirubinemia due to blood type incompatibilities (ABO or Rh) may be associated with severe anemias requiring red blood cell transfusions. (Note that we rarely transfuse whole blood—for the treatment of anemia, we would be giving so-called "packed red blood cells" [PRBCs]).

What is the prognosis in newborn jaundice?

Most premature babies with jaundice due to liver enzymes' immaturity will resolve this problem over time and their future quality of life will not be affected by it. Very few babies will have the most severe form of jaundice that progresses very quickly or reaches extremely high bilirubin levels that become toxic to the baby's brain. These conditions are called "acute bilirubin encephalopathy" and "chronic bilirubin induced neurologic dys-function" and are rare.

Part 2: Cholestatic jaundice (direct hyperbilirubinemia)

Cholestatic jaundice is diagnosed by detecting increased lev-els of "direct bilirubin" in the blood. Anatomical abnormalities in the liver, genetic conditions, infections, or prolonged use of IV nutrition can all be causes. Cholestatic jaundice due to pro-longed IV nutrition is a common occurrence among the tiniest and sickest premature babies in a NICU. Data tells us that up to 50% of babies with a birth weight of less than 1,000 grams will develop cholestatic jaundice after prolonged hyperalimentation. "Hyperalimentation" and "total parenteral nutrition (TPN)" are other names for IV nutrition. Tiny babies who suffer from multiple complications, including infections and necrotizing enterocolitis, require IV nutrition for a long time and are there-fore at risk of developing cholestatic jaundice.

Diagnosing cholestatic jaundice is easy. We use a blood test to show increased levels of "direct bilirubin." We may suspect the condition if we note on physical examination that the baby has yellowish–greenish skin. It is customary that all newborn babies receiving IV nutrition are screened for this condition once or twice a week.

We do not know the exact reasons for cholestatic jaundice. We suspect that some chemicals in IV solutions and lack of feed-ings are contributory factors. If unresolved, the condition may lead to compromised liver function and severe consequences in the future. However, the good news is that, when oral feedings are restarted and TPN is discontinued, improvement occurs within 1 to 3 months without long-term sequelae.

We have three medications at our disposal that can improve cholestatic jaundice while awaiting natural resolution. Phenobarbital is a well-known medication for seizures, but it can also be used to stimulate liver enzymes and treat cholestatic jaundice in premature babies. Ursodiol is naturally occurring bile acid. When given to babies, it improves bile flow. Finally, cholestyramine can bind bile acids in the intestines and increase their excretion from the body. All three medications can be used in combination with each other: they help but do not entirely cure cholestatic jaundice. Only the introduction of oral feedings and discontinuation of IV nutrition will allow for the complete resolution of direct hyperbilirubinemia.

CHAPTER 11

Bronchopulmonary dysplasia

Respiratory problems are widespread in premature babies. In the first few days, many develop respiratory distress syndrome (RDS; see Chapter 8). Some babies recover from RDS within days or weeks, but some never fully recover and their condition evolves into chronic lung disease called "bronchopulmonary dysplasia," or "BPD."

BPD is a pulmonary condition that develops in babies born before 32 weeks but mostly in those below 28 weeks of gestational age at birth. Because of the disruption to the lungs' proper growth and development, babies develop chronic dependence on oxygen even after overcoming the acute phase of respiratory distress after birth. Some doctors and parents use another term to describe this condition: "chronic lung disease," or "CLD."

Newborns affected by BPD will need supplementary oxygen to breathe for many weeks, months, and sometimes even more than a year. There are numerous scientific definitions of BPD used by researchers. However, the simplest one is "the need for additional oxygen to breathe at 28 days of life and/or at a corrected age of 36 weeks after birth." The most significant factor contributing to BPD's incidence is gestational age at birth (the lower the gestational age at birth, the higher the frequency of BPD).

How common is bronchopulmonary dysplasia?

Just by glancing at Table 1, it is evident that BPD, both mild and severe forms, is more common among the most premature babies, such as micro-preemies (born below 26 weeks of gestational age). Among babies born at 24 weeks, 37% will have severe BPD and 70% will have mild BPD; among 28-weekers, only 8% will have severe BPD and 24% mild BPD.

Table 1: Incidence of bronchopulmonary dysplasia (BPD) based on gestational age at birth. Mild BPD means the need for supplementary oxygen at 36 weeks of corrected age. Severe BPD means the need for treatment with more than 30% oxygen and a continuous positive airway pressure (CPAP) device or mechanical ventilation (modified from data provided by the National Institute of Child Health and Human Development network)[1].

Gestational age at birth	Mild BPD	Severe BPD
23 weeks	63%	37%
24 weeks	70%	30%
25 weeks	56%	25%
26 weeks	45%	18%
27 weeks	35%	15%
28 weeks	24%	8%

[1] *Neonatal Outcomes of Extremely Preterm Infants From the NICHD Neonatal Research Network*, Barbara J. Stoll et al. for the Eunice Kennedy Shriver National Institute of Child Health and Human Development Neonatal Research Network, Pediatrics, Sep 2010, 126 (3) 443–456; DOI: 10.1542/peds.2009-2959.

What are the risk factors for developing bronchopulmonary dysplasia?

1. <u>Prematurity</u>: I have presented data in Table 1 to show how lower gestational age at birth is associated with higher frequency of BPD in newborn babies.

2. <u>The small size of the baby at birth</u>: (Babies who are born small compared with their peers are often called "small for gestational age" or as having "intrauterine growth restriction.") One study has shown that smaller babies have a double risk of developing BPD compared with their normally grown peers.

3. <u>A mother with a history of smoking cigarettes</u>: There was a small study published that found an almost twice higher risk of BPD for babies of mothers who smoked cigarettes.

4. <u>The need for mechanical ventilation beyond seven days of life</u> (i.e. the baby receiving respiratory support on a breathing machine or ventilator): There is no doubt among neonatologists that prolonged use of mechanical ventilation is associated with a higher frequency of BPD. However, we still do not know for sure whether this is only an association or whether there is a cause–effect relationship. We continue debating what kind of respiratory support is best for babies so that we can minimize damage to the lungs and prevent the development of BPD. At this time, it appears that it is beneficial for babies to avoid mechanical ventilation if possible and to use continuous positive airway pressure (CPAP) respiratory support instead. If mechanical ventilation is necessary, some doctors advocate using volume-controlled ventilation rather than pressure-controlled (current ventilators can control both parameters if needed).

5. <u>The need for supplementary oxygen after 14 days of life</u>: We know that high concentrations of oxygen are damaging to the lungs. Unfortunately, it may be hard to avoid

giving a baby supplementary oxygen after birth if they are born with severe acute respiratory distress due to premature lungs. Also, we do not precisely know what concentrations and duration of treatment with oxygen are harmful to babies.

6. Patent ductus arteriosus (PDA; see Chapter 14): Ductus arteriosus is a vessel that, in fetal life, connects two large arteries that come out of the heart: the aorta and pulmonary arteries. After birth, in term babies, ductus arteriosus closes on its own and does not allow blood flow between those two arteries. However, in premature babies, especially the youngest ones, ductus arteriosus sometimes does not close and may contribute to the development of BPD. Many doctors have conflicting opinions on the role of ductus arteriosus and whether it should be closed medically or surgically in sick babies.

    Inflammation: Some studies say that chorioamnionitis (infection of the amniotic fluid sac) may increase the risks of developing BPD in a baby.

7. Infections after birth: Some newborns develop numerous infections during their stay in a neonatal intensive care unit (NICU). We observed that those babies also have higher risks of developing BPD.

8. Genetic factors: It is plausible that genetic factors make some babies more prone to developing BPD. Studies on this subject are ongoing.

Clinical features of bronchopulmonary dysplasia

The main clinical feature of BPD is the need for supplementary oxygen in a baby at 36 weeks of corrected gestational age. On physical examination, many babies will present with a faster than normal respiratory rate (tachypnea) and increased work of breathing, as manifested by the presence of retractions. A baby has retractions if we observe sinking chest movements in the lower ribs area while the baby is inhaling air (during inspiration).

Depending on the severity of BPD, in addition to supplementary oxygen, the baby may need to be placed on a ventilator, CPAP device, or nasal cannula. If we check the baby's blood and measure the amount of oxygen and carbon dioxide, we will often find a lower level of oxygen and increased carbon dioxide (the test is called "blood gases").

In cases where the baby needs only a small amount of extra oxygen to breathe, we can conduct a "physiologic room air trial": we will turn oxygen down to 21%, which is an amount ordinarily present in room air and follow the baby's oxygen saturation (this is a percentage of hemoglobin bound to the oxygen and can be measured easily using a monitor.) If oxygen saturation remains above 90% for at least 1 hour, the baby passes the test. This means that they probably do not need supplementary oxygen and do not meet the criteria for the diagnosis of BPD. If on room air, oxygen saturation drops below 90%, the baby should be treated with oxygen and most likely has BPD. Obviously, one should consider other clinical conditions that can also present with low blood oxygen levels.

Management and treatment of bronchopulmonary dysplasia

Most patients affected by BPD gradually improve over time. Physiologic healing processes take place as a baby is gaining weight and growing. Treatment of BPD should focus on the following areas: supporting growth, supporting work of breathing and providing oxygen if needed, and diagnosing complications.

Supporting the growth of the baby

I always tell parents that the best treatment for BPD is to make sure that the baby is gaining weight well. To achieve optimal weight gain while limiting excessive amounts of fluid volume, we have to utilize high-caloric density formulas or fortify breast milk. Pediatric dieticians advise us on adding certain additives to the baby's diet. They will also set goals for ideal weight gain in the baby (usually 20 to 30 grams per day). We do not want to achieve significant weight gain too quickly because that will be due to fluid overload, and may worsen BPD and increase oxygen requirements.

Medical treatment of bronchopulmonary dysplasia

There are several medicines that neonatologists can use for the treatment of BPD. However, there are many conflicting opinions about their utility. Many in the medical community argue that the medicines were not adequately studied and were not proved to work.

Because of a lack of better solutions, all neonatologists use at least some of these medicines in their practice. I describe these therapeutic options here without getting into controversial viewpoints:

1. Diuretics (medicines to increase urine output): It is believed that an increased amount of retained fluid in the lungs contributes to BPD. Therefore, diuretics may help in the absorption and excretion of the fluid from the lungs. Babies placed on diuretics may develop electrolyte abnormalities and may have problems with weight gain. It is crucial to monitor various metabolic parameters while we treat a patient with diuretics.
2. Caffeine: This is a medication used to treat apnea of prematurity by increasing respiratory drive. It also has diuretic effects and therefore may help in BPD.
3. Inhaled corticosteroids: Steroids decrease inflammation in the lungs. Because lung inflammation is a contributing mechanism to BPD's severity, some believe that inhaled steroids may help in its treatment.
4. Orally or intravenously administered steroids (also called "systemic steroids"): We do know that systemic steroids may facilitate quicker resolution of BPD and faster

weaning off the ventilator and oxygen. However, because of the likely adverse effects of systemic steroids on the central nervous system leading to cerebral palsy, we have to use systemic steroids very judiciously.

5. Inhaled bronchodilators (medicines used in older patients to treat asthma): Some newborns develop lung inflammation and wheezing due to spasm of the muscles located in the lower airways (bronchioles). A similar situation occurs in older patients diagnosed with asthma. Whenever we suspect such bronchospasm in a baby, we can try inhaled bronchodilators and watch whether the baby reacts positively to such a trial.

Supporting respiratory efforts

Depending on the severity of BPD, a baby may need to be placed or kept on a ventilator, CPAP device, or nasal cannula:

1. A ventilator is a machine that provides artificial and external breaths for the baby by pushing air under pressure through the tube placed in the baby's windpipe. Computer software coordinates external breaths with the baby's breathing efforts.
2. A CPAP device provides a continuous flow of air with extra pressure, particularly during the expiratory phase. This technique's primary role is to support the baby during expirations and prevent the lowest airways and alveoli from collapsing. The alveoli are the tinniest airspaces in the lungs where gas exchange takes place.
3. A nasal cannula is a small, soft, and flexible plastic tube placed in the baby's nose that provides a flow of air with oxygen.

All these three types of respiratory support can provide the desired amount of oxygen ranging from 21% up to 100%. The most advanced devices contain computer software that continuously monitors and adjusts oxygen supply to the baby's changing needs without a bedside nurse's involvement. This technology is very new and not available in all NICUs yet.

Monitoring for and treating complications of BPD

Babies suffering from BPD may develop numerous complications. Surveillance and treatment of these conditions is crucial to facilitate the path to a speedy recovery and discharge from a NICU. Let's learn about a few of them:

1. Acquired infections: Any unexpected deterioration in clinical condition may be due to an infection. Performing culture tests and treating infections with antibiotics are often necessary.

2. Air leaks (pneumothorax and pneumomediastinum): Sometimes a small portion of the lung ruptures due to air trapping and increased intrathoracic pressure. This situation may result in sudden deterioration of respiratory status and a significantly increased need for supplementary oxygen. A physical examination and chest x-ray will be diagnostic. The treatment of air leaks often involves the insertion of a needle or tube into the chest cavity to evacuate free air.

3. Systemic high blood pressure: Up to 50% of babies with BPD will also suffer from high blood pressure and will require medical treatment.

4. Fluid overload: Some babies with chronic lung disease do not tolerate a large volume of fluids and start gaining weight too rapidly with concomitant deterioration in their respiratory status. A chest x-ray will show retained fluid in their lungs. Treatment relies on fluid restriction and administration of diuretics (medications used to increase urine output).

5. Pulmonary hypertension and cor pulmonale. To diagnose this, we need to perform an ultrasound of the heart

(an "echo") and involve cardiologists. The treatment of pulmonary hypertension is long and complicated but can be successful.

Outcomes — short- and long-term outcomes

Most newborns with BPD recover from it within 2 to 4 months after diagnosis. However, babies with severe chronic lung disease may need ventilatory support and a high oxygen concentration beyond 6 months of age. Studies conducted on children of secondary- and high-school age with a diagnosis of BPD during their NICU stay have showed persistent pulmonary function abnormalities. Even though the children were not dependent on oxygen any more, they showed more airway hyperactivity (asthma-like behavior) or hyperinflation during the tests.[2] As expected, the most persistent pulmonary function abnormalities were found among survivors who had the most severe and prolonged forms of BPD.

How we can prevent bronchopulmonary dysplasia?

There are specific strategies that we can employ to prevent or mitigate the severity of BPD:

1. Preventing premature labor: Providing appropriate prenatal care and treating women at risk may delay early labor, thus decreasing the burden of prematurity.
2. Treating women in premature labor with betamethasone intramuscular injections may decrease the severity of initial respiratory disease in a baby, thus reducing the need for more invasive respiratory support such as mechanical ventilation.

---

[2] Statement on the Care of the Child with Chronic Lung Disease of Infancy and Childhood. Am J Respir Crit Care Med; 2003 Aug 1;168(3):356-96.

3. If a baby is on mechanical ventilation, using a gentler form of ventilation such as the volume-controlled mode may decrease the baby's risk of developing BPD.
4. Ensuring the ideal nutrition of the baby from the beginning will facilitate the proper growth of the lungs and allow physiologic healing mechanisms in the lungs to occur.
5. Diligent surveillance for infections and prompt treatment will eliminate additional risks for BPD.

Questions to ask your doctors if your baby has bronchopulmonary dysplasia

1. How severe is BPD in my baby?
2. What concentration of oxygen does my baby need? (The decreasing level of oxygen will be an indicator of the lungs healing. Regular room air that we all breathe in contains 21% of oxygen.)
3. How do you plan to treat my baby's chronic lung disease?
4. Do you expect that my baby will need supplementary oxygen after discharge home?
5. If I am willing to take my baby home on oxygen, will my baby go home sooner?
6. Is there anything that I can do for my baby to facilitate earlier recovery and discharge home?

CHAPTER 12

Nutrition—fluids and feedings

I n the first few days of life, many premature babies are very sick and unstable. During that time, we do everything we can to stabilize them. We often place them on a ventilator, provide supplemental oxygen, and start them on intravenous (IV) fluids. However, once this very critical period is over, the key to their continued recovery will be nutrition. Premature babies need to grow. We must provide them with enough calories and all necessary nutrients, including minerals and vitamins. Appropriate and consistent weight gain will be the best way to full recovery and discharge home.

In this chapter, I will focus on three topics: IV nutrition, the introduction of enteral feedings (using tubes and bottles), and the importance of breastmilk.

Intravenous nutrition (fluids)

Your baby is likely to require IV fluids in three scenarios: during the stabilization period (first few days of life), after we started feedings but did not reach optimal volume, and whenever your baby develops severe complications such as necrotizing entero-colitis (NEC) or infection, or needs surgery. After birth, we try to establish IV access as soon as possible to provide hydration and glucose solution to your baby. In the tiniest babies, we will insert a central line such as an umbilical catheter (UVC) or a peripherally inserted central catheter (PICC) (see Chapter 20). Because of the size of premature babies and the need for highly concentrated IV solutions, getting and maintaining regular peripheral IV access is always a challenge. Therefore, many babies born below 32 weeks, and most babies born below 28 weeks, will have a central catheter inserted. "Central" means that the tip of the catheter will be placed in a large vessel near the heart. We can obtain central IV access through the umbilicus, via a peripheral vein puncture on the hand or leg, or, as a last resort, surgically.

While providing IV nutrition, we strive to mimic the composition of the human diet. We want to include all food ingredients: sugars, proteins, fats, minerals, microelements, and vitamins. In doctors' speak, this complete IV nutrition is called "hyperalimentation" (HAL), "hyperal" or "total parenteral nutrition" (TPN). In most nurseries, trained pharmacists will calculate the exact composition of HAL solutions and order necessary blood tests needed to monitor tolerance and adverse effects.

Electrolytes (mineral) abnormalities are the most common problems while on TPN, but they are easy to fix by adjusting components of HAL solutions. Another more severe complication of IV nutrition is cholestatic jaundice, but this mostly affects babies exposed to IV nutrition for more than 2 weeks. I explained this condition in more detail in Chapter 10).

Enteral feedings (tubes and bottles)

No matter how sophisticated the IV solutions we use are, milk is the best type of nutrition for every baby. Ideally, it should be breast milk, but in some cases we are forced to use baby formulas. I will talk in more detail about breastmilk later in the chapter.

First, let's talk about different baby formulas and the actual process of feeding.

Neonatologists strongly believe that all premature babies should be receiving breastmilk. However, in cases where the mother is unable to, or does not want to, provide breastmilk, and we can't obtain donor breastmilk from a milk bank, we will use neonatal formula. Numerous formulas from different companies are suitable for premature babies. Therefore, the choice of milk will depend on parents' wishes and doctors' recommendations. There are significant differences between milk formulas for premature babies and those for term newborns. The milk for growing premature babies needs to have more protein, fat, and mineral elements, and it will be called a "high caloric density" formula. The one used has anywhere from 22 cal/oz to 30 cal/oz, while the formula for term babies has 20 cal/oz.

The digestive system in premature babies is anatomically and functionally immature. Bowel loops are shorter and smaller, and the ability to digest and absorb the milk's ingredients is diminished. Furthermore, the critical skill of drinking milk is not developed or, at best, not perfected yet. The process of drinking milk consists of three phases that need to be well coordinated:

- Sucking on the nipple or the mother's breast.
- Swallowing the liquid.
- Coordinating the sucking and swallowing with breathing, so that the milk does not enter the lungs.

Newborn babies start learning how to drink milk around 32 to 34 weeks of gestational age. For most, it is a long journey. Initially, the baby may be able to take 5 ml of milk by mouth and the rest has to be given by tube. Unless the baby is showing interest in oral feedings early, we wait to introduce bottle feedings until our patient reaches the corrected age of around 32 weeks. Until then, we provide milk to the baby using a small flexible plastic tube placed in the stomach. The tube inserted through the nose is called an "NG-tube" (nasogastric tube) and the one placed through the mouth is called an "OG-tube" (orogastric tube); either one can be used for feedings. Newborns tolerate the placement of NG/OG tubes very well, and we don't have to repeat the procedure every day because they can be left in place for several days.

Tube feedings

In stable babies, we will start these "gavage" feedings during the first few days of life. If the baby is very tiny and critically ill, we may wait much longer. The first feeding is always small and would be inadequate to provide enough calories for the baby, thus the need for IV nutrition from the very beginning. If the baby tolerates feedings well, we increase the volume of each feeding by a little bit every day until IV fluids are not needed any more. Regular stools, lack of vomiting, soft and not-distended abdomen, and weight gain are signs of an excellent feeding tolerance. If the baby develops vomiting, abdominal distension, irregular stools, or bloody stools, these are signs of feeding intolerance. In such a case, we may need to stop feedings entirely or decrease the amount of milk being provided during each feeding session. Sometimes, we can also try giving the same amount of milk but over a more extended time. For example, if today, we were giving 10 ml of milk over 20 minutes, next time we could try giving the same amount of liquid over 60 minutes. It may help babies who have intestinal peristalsis problems and a longer stomach emptying time.

From the very beginning, if a baby has a "suck reflex," we want to provide an opportunity for *non-nutritive suckling* on a pacifier during tube feedings. While milk is going directly into the stomach via a tube, the baby can practice coordinating its sucking and breathing without being in danger of aspiration. Sucking while receiving the food is also likely to stimulate specific hormones and enzymes helpful while digesting milk.

I am sure you want to know how long your baby will need an NG-tube for feedings. The answer differs. First of all, we do not know the exact answer to this question. Some babies will be able to eat everything by mouth by 36 to 37 weeks of corrected age (3 to 4 weeks before your due date). For others, it will be much longer. If your baby develops bronchopulmonary dysplasia or intraventricular hemorrhage and cannot bottle feed by 44 to 48 weeks of corrected age, they may be a candidate for a G-tube placement.

A gastrostomy tube or G-tube

Rarely, some premature babies never learn and achieve full ability to eat by mouth (using a bottle). This scenario may take place in patients with the following problems:

1. Congenital anomalies affecting the mouth, esophagus, stomach, or bowel loops.
2. Feeding problems due to extreme prematurity, neuromuscular issues, or cerebral palsy.
3. Severe motor developmental delay.

If the above situation applies to your baby and they could be ready to go home, doctors may decide to insert a G-tube so it would be easier to feed them. The G-tube is a tube inserted through the abdomen directly into the stomach. It is attached to and secured within the baby's abdominal wall. Unlike NG- or OG-tubes, the G-tube can be used for a prolonged time. It is a reasonable approach in patients who are not likely to learn within the next few weeks or months how to eat an adequate amount of food by mouth.

Breastmilk and breastfeeding

Years of research have shown that breastmilk has many benefits for the baby, mother, and even society. Due to breastfeeding, children and mothers become healthier, and society saves a significant amount of money on their care. Data proves that infants fed with breastmilk have a lower incidence of many acute and chronic pediatric diseases. The list of positively influenced conditions includes otitis media, severe diarrhea, lower respiratory tract illness, sudden infant death syndrome, inflammatory bowel disease, childhood leukemia, diabetes mellitus, obesity, asthma, and atopic dermatitis.[3]

Even more importantly, breastmilk affects premature babies very positively as well. The most important to us—neonatologists—is its effect on feeding tolerance and prevention of necrotizing enterocolitis (NEC). This is a severe complication in small premature babies that may require surgery and can lead to death (more about NEC in Chapter 13). Newborn babies who are receiving breastmilk exclusively as their diet may reach a 77% reduction in NEC incidence compared with babies receiving cows' milk-based formulas.

Other better health outcomes that have been reported in premature babies mostly fed breastmilk include:

- lower rates of retinopathy of prematurity;
- better vision;
- lower rates of infections in the neonatal intensive care unit (NICU);
- lower mortality among sick premature babies;
- shorter hospitalizations in the NICU;
- better psychomotor development.

I hope I've given you enough motivation—if you are a mother—to provide breastmilk for your baby. Unfortunately, babies born at fewer than 32 weeks are unlikely to be able to nurse. Many factors contribute to this. For one, your baby may need respiratory support (a ventilator or a continuous positive airway pressure [CPAP] device) for a long time, and therefore will not be able to eat by mouth. Second, babies born that early lack suck–swallow–breathing coordination and their first

---

[3] Evid Rep Technol Assess (Full Rep). 2007 Apr;(153):1-186. Breastfeeding and maternal and infant health outcomes in developed countries.

feedings are usually given via an NG- or OG-tube. The best way to overcome all this is to have the mother pump breastmilk so we can give it to her baby via the tube from the very first feeding. If the baby's mother can't provide breastmilk, we can obtain it from milk banks (donated breastmilk).

Pumping breastmilk

Pumping may seem challenging at first but, once you master it, it can be a very effective way to ensure adequate amounts of breastmilk for your baby. Make sure to get an electric hospital-grade breast pump. There are many available on the market and some are better suited for mothers of premature babies, so it would be best for you if you can get recommendations from lactation specialists in the NICU.

Start pumping as soon as possible, ideally no later than 4 to 6 hours after your baby's birth. Initially, you may not be able to get any milk expressed. This is completely normal: do not panic. Your body does not know that you have had a baby. The physiologic mechanisms and hormonal preparation that occur during term labor did not take place in your body. That is why you have to start pumping early and continue regularly every 2 to 3 hours, even if you are not getting any milk.

While providing breastmilk for your baby, ask for instructions on the collection, labeling, and storage of the breastmilk. Each NICU has its own policies. Below, I have included general guidelines for you:

- Review your medical history and medications with the NICU staff to make sure that breastmilk is safe for your baby.
- Obtain appropriate containers and labels from the NICU where your baby is being treated.
- Always wash your hands before touching any equipment.
- Make sure that you read the instructions and perfect the assembly of the breast pump.

- Start pumping early after the birth of your baby and continue every 2 to 3 hours. Breastfed babies typically eat every 2 to 3 hours, and your body needs to know that.
- Pumping each breast for 10 to 15 minutes is usually enough.
- It is preferable to pump both breasts simultaneously, because this stimulates higher levels of prolactin hormone, thereby helping milk production.
- When you pump, try to do it in a relaxing environment, sitting next to your baby or imagining that you are holding them. Having a Kangaroo Care session with your baby before pumping may be very helpful (see Chapter 7).
- A collection kit must be appropriately sized for your breast to optimize milk expression, and to avoid nipple trauma and pain. Some breast pumps have shield inserts to adjust the flange to your breast and nipple size.
- Most lactation experts agree that breastmilk can be stored in the refrigerator for up to 4 days and in the freezer for no more than 6 months. Containers in which you store milk need to be cleaned and labeled.
- If you have problems with your milk supply, ask your baby's neonatologist whether you should try a herb called "fenugreek" or a medication—Reglan. Both are believed to increase breastmilk supply.

Breastmilk from the bank (human donor milk)

Neonatologists and pediatric organizations consider breastmilk to be a necessary treatment for premature babies born with a birthweight of fewer than 1,500 grams. We recommend using human donor milk for families in which the mother is unable to provide breastmilk. In the USA and many Western countries, donor breastmilk is pasteurized and comes from private and public milk banks. Medical professionals caution us against buying human milk on the internet or getting it from friends. If you do that, you have a higher risk of obtaining a contaminated or infected product.

Pasteurization methods used by the milk banks are able to eliminate from breastmilk viruses HIV, cytomegalovirus, Hepatitis B and C, and bacteria. In my opinion, donor breastmilk has many more benefits than risks. However, if you are worried about unknown exposure from donors of milk to drugs, medications, or herbs, you should discuss it with your baby's neonatologist.

You can learn more about human donor milk from the Human Milk Banking Association of North America at www.HMBANA.com and the Prolacta Bioscience at www.prolacta.com.

Milk fortifiers

Maternal breastmilk will typically have no more than 20 cal/oz (20 cal/30 ml). On the other hand, premature babies need more calorie-dense milk to grow. That forces us to add extra liquid or powder to breastmilk to achieve optimal caloric intake. We call these products "fortifiers" or "human milk fortifiers," and, when using them, we can achieve milk caloric density ranging from 22 cal/oz to 30 cal/oz. You may ask: why can't we give more milk to your baby instead of making it thicker? That is a good question, but there is a limit to the amount of fluid we can safely give your baby each day. If we gave too much liquid, we would facilitate more chronic breathing problems or patent ductus arteriosus. Deciding about types of feedings for the baby involves finding a balance between the volume of fluids we can provide and the number of calories needed for growth.

CHAPTER 13

Necrotic enterocolitis

N ecrotic enterocolitis (NEC) is a severe abdominal condition affecting mostly extremely premature babies and
micro-preemies. It usually occurs 2 weeks or later after
birth and may result in long-lasting adverse consequences for
the baby, or even death. After a tiny baby overcomes initial acute
respiratory distress after birth, diseases such as NEC, bronchopulmonary dysplasia (BPD), retinopathy of prematurity (ROP) and
infections may negatively affect their well-being. After 2 weeks
of age, NEC and infections are the most likely to be the cause of
death for babies in a neonatal intensive care unit (NICU).

Definition of necrotic enterocolitis
and background information

NEC is a severe abdominal condition that affects the gastrointestinal tract in a newborn baby. The disease's actual mechanism
and etiology are poorly understood, but we believe that several
processes play a role in its development:

- Decreased blood flow to the bowel loops.
- Necrosis (death) of the intestinal lining (= intestinal mucosa).

- Inflammation in the intestines.
- Microorganisms entering the intestinal lining and sometimes the blood vessels.
- The gas produced by microorganisms entering the intestinal walls and blood vessels.
- Rupture of the bowel loops' walls and a severe infection in the abdominal cavity called "peritonitis."

Incidence

Ninety percent of NEC cases occur in premature babies, and only about 10% in full-term babies. The incidence of NEC in babies born at fewer than 32 weeks of gestational age varies from 2% to 7%. The frequency of the disease increases with decreasing gestational age at birth and lower birth weight. Micro-preemies are the most affected group of babies (see Tables 13.1 and 13.2).

Table 13.1: Incidence rates including all types of necrotic enterocolitis (stages 1–3). Adapted from "National prospective surveillance study of necrotizing enterocolitis in neonatal intensive care units." Journal of Pediatric Surgery 45(7):1391-7 July 2010

Gestational age at birth	Incidence of necrotic enterocolitis
Fewer than 26 weeks	14%
26–28 weeks	10.8%
28–32 weeks	3%

Table 13.2: Adapted from "Effect of deregionalized care on mortality in very low-birth-weight infants with necrotizing enterocolitis." JAMA Pediatr. 2015 Jan;169(1):26-32

Birth weight	Incidence of necrotic enterocolitis
Fewer than 1,000 grams	9.4%
1,000–1,499 grams	3.9%

Diagnosing necrotic enterocolitis

Whenever doctors suspect NEC in a baby, they will review clinical symptoms, perform imaging studies of the abdomen, and do some laboratory tests.

Often, the first sign of NEC is the development of feeding intolerance. Premature newborns will have increased gastric residuals after tube feedings, bloody stools, and abdominal distention. When the disease becomes more advanced, babies present with increased sleepiness or lethargy, apneas (pauses in breathing), heart rate drops, abdominal tenderness, and discoloration of the skin on the abdomen. The sickest babies will also have temperature instability and abnormally low blood pressure, which are often signs of overwhelming infection (sepsis) and a bowel perforation.

We can use an abdominal x-ray and abdominal ultrasound to aid us in the diagnosis of NEC. However, an abdominal x-ray remains the most popular technique.

Pneumatosis (presence of air within the bowel walls) is diagnostic if found on an abdominal x-ray of a baby suspected of having NEC.

Other radiologic (x-ray) findings in NEC include:

- ileus—lack of peristalsis or intestinal movements;
- dilated intestines;
- presence of air in the portal vein (a blood vessel in the liver);
- free air in the abdominal cavity that is a result of ruptured bowel loops.

Abdominal ultrasound allows doctors to evaluate the presence of fluid, the thickness of the intestinal walls, and blood flow to the intestines. Ultrasound is a less popular method of assessing babies with NEC because it requires more experience from the examiner.

Laboratory tests are an essential part of the diagnostic process for detecting NEC. The most commonly conducted tests are blood cultures, blood counts, and coagulation studies.

Blood cultures are done to confirm or rule out the presence of bacterial infections. A positive result will allow us to choose the best antibiotics for the treatment.

Complete blood counts (CBCs) in babies with NEC will often show anemia, low or high white cell counts and low platelet levels. These abnormalities are not specific only to the NEC diagnosis but can support our suspicion of it in the patient.

Coagulation studies look at levels of relevant clotting factors in the blood. In the sickest babies diagnosed with NEC, these indices will be abnormal and may require plasma or platelet transfusions to correct them.

Staging severity of NEC

In the effort to describe different presentations and prognoses in NEC, clinicians classify each case into one of the following three categories:

Stage 1: Suspected NEC (mild NEC)
Babies have abdominal distention, bloody stools, and vomiting or gastric residuals. On x-ray, we will see signs of ileus and bowel loops dilation.

Stage 2: Proven NEC (moderate NEC)
Clinically, the baby will present with abdominal tenderness. Laboratory tests will show acidosis (more acid in the blood) and low platelet counts. An x-ray will show pneumatosis and/or the presence of gas in the portal vein.

Stage 3: Advanced NEC (severe NEC)
In addition to previously described clinical features, the baby is also likely to have low blood pressure, low white cell counts, low platelet counts, and significant acidosis. An x-ray in advanced NEC will show ruptured bowel loops with free air in the abdominal cavity.

Can my baby have something other than necrotizing enterocolitis?

As with any other medical diagnosis, whenever we make a diagnosis of NEC, we need to consider other diagnoses to avoid mistakes. I describe here some of the conditions that may mislead us into thinking that your baby has NEC:

1. Anal fissure: Babies with anal fissure may present with bloody stools, and we know that bloody stools may occur in NEC as well.
2. Milk allergy: This is a rare occurrence in a baby before 6 to 8 weeks of age, but sometimes it can happen, particularly in babies fed with formula. Affected babies may have abdominal distention, frequent stools, and bloody stools.
3. Overwhelming infection or sepsis: Babies with an ongoing infectious disease may present with apnea, low blood pressure, and feeding intolerance, including ileus on abdominal x-ray.
4. Spontaneous intestinal perforation: This is a sporadic condition. It may occur in babies born with birth weights below 1,500 grams. The differentiation from NEC is that there will be no pneumatosis (air in the intestinal wall) on the x-ray.
5. Appendicitis: Another rare condition in newborns that may lead to perforation and infection in the abdominal cavity (peritonitis).
6. Viral or bacterial enteritis: Infection of the gastro-enteric tract may present itself with abdominal distention, frequent stools, bloody stools, and deterioration of the general condition.

How do we treat NEC?

There is no specific treatment for NEC. Our approach will vary depending on the severity of the condition and will involve multiple steps described below.

Supportive care

Babies with diagnosed or suspected NEC will not receive any feedings (we say that they are to be NPO ["nil per os", "nothing by mouth"]). In addition, we often place a large plastic tube in their stomach and connect it to intermittent suction to remove gas from the abdomen and allow the bowel loops to rest. Most babies will not be receiving any milk by mouth for 10 to 14 days. Therefore, we place a central intravenous line so that we can give them appropriate fluids and nutrition. Many newborns with NEC need to be placed on ventilators with supplementary oxygen, receive medications to support their blood pressure, and given transfusions of blood products.

Empiric antibiotics

Empiric use of antibiotics in the treatment of NEC is a must. Approximately 30% of babies diagnosed with NEC will have positive blood cultures, which means that they will have actual bacteria identified in their blood. In remaining patients, bacterial overgrowth in the intestines is likely to damage the intestinal mucosa, leading to local inflammation. Therefore, the use of antibiotics is also wise.

Close monitoring

NEC is always an evolving condition and may get much worse very quickly. Doctors monitor all babies carefully to detect early changes in their health and acute complications requiring changes in the treatment approach.

Monitoring almost always will include:

- frequent physical examinations with abdominal girth measurements (a stable or decreasing abdominal circumference is a positive sign);
- regular abdominal x-rays (some findings on x-ray may warrant urgent surgical consult and operation);
- continuous monitoring of respiratory and heart rates, blood pressure, and oxygen saturation (that is done using bedside monitors always present in a NICU);
- blood tests (levels of electrolytes, blood counts, and clotting factors).

Surgical procedures

Babies with the most severe form of NEC may need surgical treatment. The absolute indication for the surgical approach is a perforated bowel with free air present in the abdominal cavity. Other indications are less specific and will vary depending on the center's experience. Approximately 50% of babies with true NEC require surgical procedures.

There are two surgical techniques available: open abdomen surgery (laparotomy) and placement of the drain (Penrose drain). Surgeons and neonatologists have been studying both methods over the past decade, trying to establish which one may be better. However, this question has not yet been answered adequately. It seems that both approaches have similar rates of death and complications, but studied sample sizes have not been big enough to say that with certainty.

1. *Laparotomy or open abdomen surgery:* The baby needs to be put under general anesthesia. A surgeon cuts through all the layers of the abdominal wall, cleans the abdominal cavity, resects dead pieces of the bowel loops, and usually creates an ostomy. An ostomy is an opening in the abdomen created by the surgeon to allow intestinal contents

to come out. In NEC, the purpose of an ostomy is to let the rest of the bowel loops heal and recover over time. Once the baby recovers from the NEC and the bowel loops are healed, they will need further surgery to close the intestines' ostomy and return continuity so that stools can be expelled through the anus again.

2. *Penrose drain*: This method is the only one that we offer to babies who are too unstable to undergo surgery under general anesthesia. Penrose drain placement can be done using only local anesthesia at the bedside. A surgeon can place a Penrose drain under local anesthesia in the NICU instead of the operating room. The Penrose drain is a small tubing that can be put into the abdominal cavity. The goal is to decompress the abdomen and to irrigate and drain out infectious contents. If the baby survives the acute phase of NEC, the Penrose drain is removed and doctors evaluate the baby's gastrointestinal tract to ensure that they can safely start feedings.

Outcomes in babies with a diagnosis of NEC

Despite many improvements in the care of babies affected by NEC, it is still a condition associated with significant mortality and many short-term and long-term complications. Also, survivors tend to have less favorable developmental outcomes than peers who do not have the NEC diagnosis.

Mortality

NEC may be responsible for up to 10% of all deaths in advanced NICUs caring for all types of premature babies. Data gathered from 655 US-based centers between 2006 and 2010 showed an overall 28% mortality for babies diagnosed with NEC. Mortality is higher for smaller and more premature babies and for those who require surgical treatment (see Table 13.3).

Table 13.3: Mortality rates for different birth weights. Data covers years 2005–06. Source: "Mortality of necrotizing enterocolitis expressed by birth weight categories." J Pediatr Surg 2009 Jun;44(6):1072-5.

Birth weight	Mortality from necrotizing enterocolitis
1,250–1,500 grams	16%
1,000–1,250 gram	21%
750–1,000 grams	29%
501–750 grams	42%

Complications

Babies affected by NEC may develop acute and chronic or long-term complications.

Potential acute problems

- Infections: Up to 30% of babies with NEC will have confirmed generalized systemic infection. Many will also develop pneumonia, peritonitis, or abscesses.
- Respiratory problems: Many babies diagnosed with NEC will have to be placed on a ventilator even if they have previously been weaned off one.
- Heart failure and low blood pressure: Some babies need medications to maintain healthy levels of blood pressure.
- Excessive bleeding: Some babies will need platelet or plasma transfusions to improve their clotting ability.
- Metabolic abnormalities in the blood: For example, acidosis, low glucose, low or high sodium levels, and many others.
- Kidney failure: due to infections, fluid imbalances, or clotting abnormalities, the baby may develop an abnormal renal function.

Long-term complications after necrotizing enterocolitis

The most important long-term complications of NEC are the conditions that can have an impact on absorption, patency, or peristalsis of the intestines:

1. Babies with NEC diagnoses will develop *strictures* in 10% to 35% of cases. Strictures are scars built of connective tissue, often compressing bowel loops from the outside, causing a narrowing, and decreasing their patency. Therefore, they may contribute to feeding intolerance and, in some cases, cause complete obstruction.

2. Short bowel syndrome: in babies with severe NEC, a surgeon may need to remove a significant portion of dead bowel loops. If the baby ends up with less than 25% of the normal intestines' length, they may develop short bowel syndrome. Babies with short bowel syndrome will have significant nutritional problems due to the inability to absorb essential nutrients from milk and, later on, from solid food. These babies are likely to be affected by many medical issues, including very poor physical growth.

3. Motor and intellectual development: infants with NEC diagnosis are at increased risk of having growth failure, cerebral palsy, intellectual disability, and vision problems. The risk of these problems may be as high as twice that for matched newborns who do not have NEC. It also seems that the severity of NEC plays a role because babies who require surgical treatment tend to have more poor outcomes than those who are treated only medically.

Prevention of necrotic enterocolitis

The most obvious way to avoid NEC is to prevent premature birth. If you are already in early labor, you may want to talk to your obstetrician as to whether you should receive Betamethasone. Steroid medications such as Betamethasone or Dexamethasone, when administered to women in premature labor at least 24 to 48 hours before the baby's actual birth, decrease rates of acute respiratory distress, mortality, intraventricular hemorrhage, ROP and NEC.

If your baby is already born and being treated in a NICU, neonatologists will try to follow specific practice guidelines that are believed to decrease rates of NEC. One approach that is probably the most powerful is to provide breastmilk to all premature babies instead of formula.

Most doctors who treat premature babies believe that the practices described below decrease rates of NEC. However, not all of them are well documented by research and evidence:

- Avoidance of prolonged antibiotic treatment courses in the NICU.
- Avoidance of use of medications that decrease acidity in the stomach (so-called "H2 blockers").
- Using feeding protocols in the NICU (being careful about daily increases in feeding volumes).
- Treatment of polycythemia (a high number of red blood cells).
- Exclusive use of breastmilk for feedings.
- Use of probiotics (still controversial in the USA).

If somebody asked me what the best medicine used in a NICU is, I would quickly answer: breastmilk. *Breastmilk is a miracle solution for premature babies.* Exclusive use of breastmilk for feedings most likely contributes to lower mortality rates, decreased infections, less NEC, and a faster discharge home from the unit. Compared with bovine protein-based formula, human milk has been shown to reduce the risk of NEC. The effect is dose-dependent, meaning that, when the higher percentage of total feeding volumes is given as breastmilk, the risk of developing NEC by the baby is lower. If a mother is unable to provide breastmilk for her baby, we can use breastmilk obtained from a breastmilk bank. Donor breastmilk also has been shown to have protective effects on the risk of NEC, and is highly recommended for micro-preemies and extremely premature babies.

Probiotics are live bacteria that can be given to babies in order to facilitate positive health outcomes, including a decrease in the rate of NEC. Despite numerous studies that have been conducted so far, many questions and concerns remain and prevent most US neonatologists from using them. Many studies have shown benefits of probiotics for mortality rates and NEC rates in newborns, but those positive results are inconsistent for the most vulnerable groups, such as micro-preemies. Also, questions remain regarding an appropriate product containing probiotics, dosage, indications for it, and treatment duration. Additional concerns are that the use of probiotics in most vulnerable patients, such as micro-preemies and extremely premature babies, may cause severe infection (sepsis).

Questions to ask if your baby is in a neonatal intensive care unit and has necrotic enterocolitis:

1. How certain are you about the NEC diagnosis?
2. Which stage of NEC does my baby have?
3. What can I do for my baby?
4. Do you have a pediatric surgeon in place so that my baby will receive optimal treatment if required?
5. If you do not have a pediatric surgeon available on site, should we transfer my baby to another institution as soon as they are stable enough to undergo such transport?
6. How long will my baby be on antibiotics?
7. How long do you expect to keep my baby NPO (without any milk for feedings)?
8. Does my baby have any acute complications due to NEC?

CHAPTER 14

Patent ductus arteriosus

P atent ductus arteriosus (PDA) is a cardiovascular condition occurring exclusively in newborn babies. When
severe, it affects other neonatal outcomes such as survival, oxygen dependence, necrotizing enterocolitis (NEC), and
long-term development. In this chapter, I will explain its definition, diagnosis, therapeutic options, and outcomes.

To understand PDA, we need to know a little bit about heart
anatomy in a fetus and the changes that occur soon after birth.
The human heart consists of four chambers: two atriums and two
ventricles. Arteries come out of the heart, and veins bring blood
back to the heart. The aorta, the largest artery, comes out of the
left ventricle and provides blood to all our organs. The pulmonary
artery comes out of the right ventricle and takes blood to the
lungs to get oxygenated. Then blood with oxygen goes back to the
left atrium through veins and subsequently leaves the heart again
through the aorta. The difference is that the lungs of a fetus are
filled with liquid, and there is no oxygen there because the fetus
(before birth) is not breathing air yet. That is why nature equipped
us with an additional vessel called a "ductus arteriosus." This vessel

connects the pulmonary artery with the aorta. In the fetus, blood leaving the heart through the pulmonary artery will pass by the lungs and go directly to the aorta via the ductus arteriosus route. After birth, once the baby starts breathing, blood from the pulmonary artery flows into the lungs to pick up oxygen, and the ductus arteriosus should stop functioning. Because of increased oxygen levels and blood pressure changes after birth, the ductus arteriosus constricts and later tissue growth completely obstructs its lumen leading to its disappearance. These changes occur in full-term newborn babies within 24 to 48 hours after birth. If the ductus arteriosus remains wide open in very premature babies, it may be associated with increased mortality, more severe lung disease (bronchopulmonary dysplasia [BPD]), and higher incidences of intraventricular hemorrhage (IVH) and NEC.

PDA incidence among babies born with a birth weight of fewer than 1,500 g (3.3 lb) is about 30%. As with any other neonatal problem, the incidence increases with decreasing birth weight and gestational age at birth. Severe respiratory disease and infections are additional contributing factors in the sickest premature babies, and they inhibit physiologic mechanisms responsible for ductal closure.

Diagnosis of patent ductus arteriosus

We may suspect PDA in a baby presenting with certain clinical features, but only by doing an "echo" (an ultrasound of the heart) can we make the ultimate diagnosis.

The following are clinical findings suggestive of PDA in a premature baby:

1. Sudden deterioration or lack of improvement in respiratory status. For example, need for higher concentration of oxygen.
2. Presence of a heart murmur on examination.
3. "Wide" blood pressures (significant difference between systolic and diastolic pressures).

4. Low blood pressure (hypotension).
5. Large heart on x-rays.
6. Decreased urine output.
7. A higher amount of acid in blood tests (= acidosis).

Some neonatologists will do an echo during the first week of life in all newborn babies born at fewer than 28 weeks of gestational age (we call it "screening for PDA"). Others will order the test only in babies who show at least some of PDA's clinical features. The echo is a relatively easy test and can be done at the bedside but it does require an experienced technician. Once done, we can send it via the internet to a cardiologist and obtain a quick reading.

The results will guide our approach to treating this condition. Therefore, we want answers to several questions:

- Is the ductus arteriosus open?
- What is the size of the PDA (more than 1.4 mm is significant)?
- Is there a blood flow via the ductus arteriosus? How much blood flow is present?
- If the flow of blood is present, is it one-directional or bi-directional? Is it from right to left or from left to right?

Treatment of patent ductus arteriosus

Neonatologists still keep arguing about whether PDA treatment is necessary and, if it is, how and when to do it. People who argue against treating this condition claim that it is just a natural feature of prematurity, and that in most cases the ductus arteriosus closes on its own although this does not happen right after birth as in full-term babies. Doctors who want to treat it bring up the counter-argument that premature babies with a moderate or large PDA have higher mortality rates than babies without it. Therefore, we can't ignore it.

As with everything in our lives, moderation is probably the best approach, and that's what most neonatal centers do. Treatment of clinically significant PDA starts with a conservative approach. Then, after some time, infants who remain on a ventilator with high settings will be treated with medications. Finally, newborns who require a ventilator with maximum support, and have failed one or two rounds of medical treatment, may be candidates for surgical closure.

The conservative approach does not mean doing nothing. Indeed, we restrict the baby's intravenous or total fluid volume, adjust respiratory support, treat anemia trying to maintain the hematocrit above 30%-35%, and use diuretics (medicines that increase urine output).

For pharmacologic closure of PDA, we can use one of three medicines available to us: Indomethacin, Ibuprofen, Acetaminophen (Ibuprofen = Advil and Acetaminophen = Tylenol). Most of you will know the last two very well because they are popular medicines used by adults for pain and fever. All three drugs have similar mechanisms of action and, if effective, they will cause constriction of the ductus arteriosus. Indomethacin and Ibuprofen are the best studied so far. Some argue that Ibuprofen is a preferable option because data indicates that it is less likely to cause specific side effects such as decreased urine output or NEC. Babies who suffer from uncontrolled infection, active bleeding, low platelets, compromised urine output, NEC, or IVH usually are not good candidates for the treatment with Ibuprofen and Indomethacin. Both medicines may worsen any condition related to increased bleeding or impaired kidney function. For those newborns, we can consider using Acetaminophen because it has a slightly different mechanism of action and profile of side effects.

If one or two rounds of pharmacologic treatment fail to close the ductus arteriosus and the baby is still on very high settings on a ventilator, we may consider a surgical approach. We can achieve surgical ligation either through open-chest surgery or via the percutaneous transcatheter occlusion (minimally invasive surgery). The choice of surgical technique will depend on the size of the baby and the surgeon's experience. However, the US Food and Drug Administration has approved a minimally invasive procedure only for newborns with a weight of more than 700 g (1.5 lb) and older than 3 days.

Outcomes in babies with patent ductus arteriosus

It has been reported that mortality among babies who develop significant PDA and fail medical closure is increased fourfold compared with newborns who have never had a clinically significant PDA. There is no difference in death rates between groups of babies with successfully treated PDA and groups of newborns without PDA at all. We also know that a large PDA is associated with higher rates of other neonatal complications such as BPD, NEC, and IVH.

The good news is that the medical treatment of PDA is quite successful and reaches desired results in up to 70% of treated babies. Furthermore, even if PDA is left alone, without any treatment, a significant number of babies undergo closure spontaneously over time.

CHAPTER 15

Heart-related problems—blood pressure, murmurs, arrhythmias

Patent ductus arteriosus (PDA) is the only cardiovascular problem directly linked to prematurity (see Chapter 14). However, premature babies undergoing treatment in a neonatal intensive care unit (NICU) must often be evaluated for other heart problems.

This chapter will focus on three types of cardiovascular problems: blood pressure, heart murmurs, and arrhythmias. You may be lucky, and your baby may never have any of these.

Blood pressure

It would be best to think about our blood vessels as a network of numerous pipes of different sizes connected to a pump cyclically pushing blood in one direction. Blood vessels are like pipes, and the heart is the pump. Blood pressure in our circulation will depend on the force of the heart contractions and resistance in blood vessels. There are many factors capable of influencing these two parameters and resulting in low blood pressure (hypotension), normal blood pressure, or high blood pressure (hypertension). Hypotension and hypertension need to be treated if significant because they may damage the brain, heart, or kidneys.

Babies who suffer from acute blood loss, develop an overwhelming infection (sepsis), or are extremely premature will often have low blood pressure. High blood pressure is more likely to occur in babies who have bronchopulmonary dysplasia, are in pain, or had umbilical catheters inserted after birth.

The good news is that we have many effective medications available to treat both hypotension and hypertension. Identifying the cause contributing to abnormal blood pressure will help in addressing and solving the problem more quickly.

Heart murmurs

A heart murmur is a noise heard by a doctor while listening to a baby's heart. It originates due to turbulent blood flow within the heart and large blood vessels. Finding a heart murmur may help diagnose an abnormality in the heart but it is by no means diagnostic. Many babies with completely normal heart anatomy and function have heart murmurs. Some say that a physician with good hearing will find heart murmurs in up to 70% of babies staying in a NICU. However, only a small fraction of them will have significant cardiovascular disease.

If doctors think that a heart murmur is suggestive of abnormal heart anatomy, they will order an echo (an ultrasound study of the heart, allowing us to assess its structure and function). An echo is a relatively straightforward study, can be performed at the bedside and takes an average of 15 to 20 minutes. It requires a skilled technician to perform it and then a pediatric cardiologist to read it. Because of modern technology, cardiologists can read it even from another location if results are needed urgently.

A heart murmur is only one of many possible symptoms suggestive of abnormal heart anatomy. Other symptoms include respiratory problems (need for extra oxygen, fast breathing), low blood pressure, difficulties with feeding, pale or cyanotic skin color, and reduced urine output. A baby with a heart murmur without any other symptoms is likely to have less severe heart disease than a baby with many other accompanying abnormal findings.

The treatment of anatomical heart abnormalities will depend on the severity and urgency of the situation. Some defects may just be watched and will resolve over time (e.g. ventricular septum defect [VSD], or patent foramen ovale [PFO]). Other heart defects may need urgent surgery. Unfortunately, if an operation is necessary, the size of the premature baby may be an obstacle: in most cases, we have a minimum weight before surgery can be performed on a baby. However, these criteria may vary depending on the center's experience.

Arrhythmias

Our hearts are supposed to contract regularly at specific frequencies that depend on our age, blood pressure, and physical activity. An adult's heart rate, at rest, is approximately 60 beats per minute. A newborn's heart rate is usually between 120 and160 per minute. A crying baby may briefly have a heart beating at 180 to 200 per minute.

Due to various factors, some babies suffer from a fast heart rate (tachycardia), a low heart rate (bradycardia), or an irregular heart rhythm (arrhythmia). Without going into too much detail, let me say that some of those conditions will have a negative impact on the blood flow to vital organs (brain, kidneys, bowels), and will require treatment.

Most of the time, heart rate problems are spotted by a nurse on a bedside cardiorespiratory monitor. While making a diagnosis, we rely on two studies: ECG (electrocardiogram) and Holter. An ECG is an electric study of the heart conducted over a short time (15 to 30 seconds). It is done by placing the leads on the baby's chest and limbs and obtaining a graph from the machine depicting the heart's electrical function. The Holter study allows us to record heart rate and all irregularities over a more extended period of time, such as 12 to 24 hours. If we suspect that a particular rhythm abnormality is due to improper heart anatomy, we will also order an Echo (ultrasound study of the heart).

The treatment of arrhythmias depends on the specific diagnosis and how much the baby is affected. In cases where blood flow to vital organs is compromised due to a very fast heart rate, we can use electric shock therapy applied directly to the chest area (defibrillation or cardioversion). Other significant but not urgent arrhythmias can be treated with medications or laser therapy. Using a laser technique, we can burn improper conduction pathways in the heart. Benign arrhythmias can be just watched, waiting for their resolution over time.

I have only given you an overview of cardiac conditions that may need to be addressed in premature babies. I have not gone into a lot of details here because it is a very complicated topic, it is not specific to premature babies, and it would probably require another book by itself!

CHAPTER 16

Retinopathy of prematurity

Retinopathy of prematurity (ROP) is a cause of anxiety for many families of micro-preemies and extremely premature babies. They fear that the condition will lead to vision problems or blindness after discharge home.

ROP is a disease of growing and proliferating blood vessels in the back of immature eyes. Premature babies are always born with immature eyes. During the first months after birth, blood vessels in the eyes must grow and multiply. Disruption of that natural process by various factors may lead to ROP.

According to ophthalmologists, ROP is one of the significant causes of blindness in the USA.

Eye anatomy

Before we go any further on the topic, let me review some general information regarding eye anatomy. If you have some knowledge about the structure and functioning of the eye, just skip this part and go to the next section.

In Figure 16.1 below, you can see that the eye is cross-cut along its anterior-posterior axis.

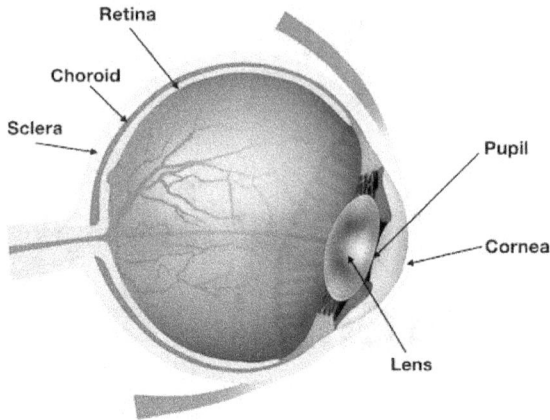

The eye is a globular structure covered by several membranes and filled with a liquid substance called "vitreous humor". It is made up of the following parts:

- Cornea: a clear and transparent dome-like structure covering the front of the eye.
- Iris: a thin, colored, circular structure that controls the size of the pupil and is located behind the cornea and in front of the lens.
- Pupil: a round opening within the iris that allows light to go inside the eye.
- Lens: a transparent structure located behind the iris and capable of bending or focusing light rays on the back of the eye where vision receptors are located.
- Retina: an internal lining of the eye filled with light-sensitive receptors. Light stimulates the receptors and produces electric signals sent through the optic nerve to the brain areas responsible for vision.

- Choroid: a membrane that lies behind the retina and supplies nutrition to the eye through blood vessels.
- Vitreous humor: a fluid that fills the eye globe between the lens and the retina.

How common is retinopathy of prematurity?

ROP occurs more frequently in the tiniest and most premature babies. Let's look at **Table 16.1** to see its incidence.

Age at birth	All types of ROP	Severe ROP
<24 weeks	95%	18%
25 weeks	92%	12%
26 weeks	85%	12%
27 weeks	72%	5%
28 weeks	66%	4%

You will notice that the more premature babies have a higher risk of developing ROP. For example, more than 90% of babies born at below 25 weeks will develop some kind of ROP, and more than 10% of them will have a severe form of it. At 28 weeks of gestational age, those numbers drop to 66% for any ROP and to 4% for severe ROP.

Researchers have identified four main risk factors associated with ROP: small birth weight, low gestational age, unmonitored oxygen use, and high glucose levels requiring insulin treatment. We also know that, if a baby needs more aggressive therapies or develops complications in a neonatal intensive care unit (NICU), such a baby will have a higher risk for ROP. Epidemiological studies tell us that babies who stay for a long time on a ventilator, have abnormal blood gases, require blood transfusion, or develop infections, pneumothorax, or intraventricular hemorrhages have a much higher chance of having ROP (*Pneumothorax* is a condition in which a portion of the lung ruptures and air leaks out of the lung and gathers in the chest, compressing the lung and preventing it from expanding. *Intraventricular hemorrhage* is a bleed in one of the brain's areas, and a complication to which very premature babies are prone).

Unmonitored exposure to high oxygen concentrations during the first weeks of life is also associated with a higher incidence of ROP. Unfortunately, the optimal way of providing oxygen to babies is still unclear to us. It appears that lower oxygenation targets are safer for the eyes. On the other hand, we know that lower oxygen levels, particularly in the smallest babies, increase deaths. At this time, most NICUs are targeting oxygen saturations in the range of 90% to 95%. Only a few doctors advocate targeting oxygen saturations below 85% because of increased mortality in the tiniest babies. Please remember that these numbers may change at any time as new data gets published.

(*Oxygen saturation* is the number obtained from the monitors, always present at the bedside, that allow us to indirectly assess oxygen levels.)

Mechanism of retinopathy of prematurity

ROP may develop in two phases. Phase 1 starts soon after birth and is defined by the arrest of blood vessels growth due to exposure to too much oxygen. The term "too much" should be understood as too much for growing blood vessels in the eye, but the same amount of oxygen is often appropriate and even necessary for the baby to survive. *I don't want anybody to think that a baby develops ROP because doctors have given too much oxygen to a baby: that is never the case.*

In Phase 1, oxygen leads to decreased production of so-called blood vessels growth factors (erythropoietin and vascular endothelial growth factor [VEGF]) and that in turn leads to the arrest of blood vessels growth.

Phase 1 may evolve into Phase 2, and that usually occurs after 32 weeks of corrected gestational age. In Phase 2, due to poorly developed blood vessels, the retina is starved of oxygen. That situation stimulates over-production of growth factors and unhealthy retinal blood vessels growth follows, resulting—in the worst scenario—in retinal detachment and blindness.

In many premature babies, the retina revascularizes properly after Phase 1 and retinal detachment does not occur. However, even after mild ROP, many babies may end up with insufficient numbers of photoreceptors (light receptors) in their eyes and will develop various vision problems later on in life.

Which premature babies should be screened for retinopathy of prematurity?

To diagnose ROP disease early and be able to start treatment to limit the negative consequences of the disease, we must screen babies for ROP. Many professional organizations state that all babies born at fewer than 30 weeks of gestational age, or with a birth weight of fewer than 1,500 g, should be regularly screened for ROP. Of course, these criteria mean that *all* micro-preemies and extremely premature babies must be screened. Most of the time, ROP screening is conducted by ophthalmologists in person. However, in some centers, it is done by technicians who use unique cameras to take pictures of the baby's eyes and send those pictures to eye-doctors for a reading. The latter approach is less desirable because it can miss some milder forms of ROP. However, because of a shortage of available eye-doctors, using a camera to conduct an ROP examination in the hospital where your baby is being cared for may be the only option.

At what age should the retinopathy of prematurity exam be done?

We don't perform screening exams for ROP until several weeks after birth. You have to remember that a baby is never born with ROP: they develop ROP over time. Based on historical statistical information, doctors decided that ROP exams should start at 30 weeks of corrected gestational age for babies born between 22 and 26 weeks, and at 4 weeks of age for babies born at 27 weeks of gestational age or more. Just be aware that individual hospitals may have a slightly different schedule and policy for these exams.

How is the retinopathy of prematurity exam conducted?

The ROP exam is done at the bedside. In preparation for the exam, eye drops are instilled to dilate the pupils, and sucrose can be given to the baby to make them more comfortable. An assistant will swaddle the baby and hold their head down while the ophthalmologist looks into their eyes using special lenses and lights. The whole exam does not take very long, probably 5 to 10 minutes, and most babies tolerate it well.

Assessing the severity of retinopathy of prematurity

After conducting the ROP exam, the ophthalmologist will assess the severity of illness individually for each eye using four descriptors: zone, stage, the extent of disease, and the presence or absence of plus disease. Let's look at the meaning of these four terms.

The zone is an area of the eye where abnormal blood vessels are found (see Figure 16.2 below). Zone 1 is the most posterior and of utmost importance because it covers the highest concentration of light receptors. Disease in zone 1 places you at the highest risk for visual acuity loss. ROP in zones 2 and 3 is less dangerous for vision loss.

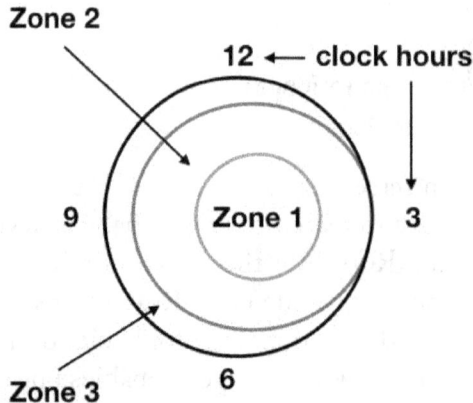

ROP stages: Based on how the blood vessels and retina look during the exam, the ophthalmologist may classify ROP disease within the range of *Stages 1 to 5*. Stage 1 is the most benign while Stage 5 signifies the most severe ROP form consistent with retinal detachment.

The disease's extent is recorded by comparing the bottom of the eye to a clock and stating how many clock hours are involved. For example, a doctor may say that ROP is present in the left eye from 1 to 4 and then from 7 to 9 clock hours.

Plus disease is present when we see tortuous blood vessels in the retina. ROP with abnormal tortuous vessels is always a more aggressive form of ROP and indicates a high risk of progression to retinal detachment.

Indications for treatment of ROP

- Any stage ROP with the plus disease in zone I.
- Stage 3 ROP without the plus disease in zone I.
- Stage 2 or 3 ROP with the plus disease in zone 2.

You may ask why we need to treat ROP if we know that the natural evolution of this disease is that it regresses, and that current treatments are not the ultimate cure for the disease. It is an excellent question. The answer is that, when we use the indications as mentioned above, there is less chance for adverse visual outcomes than if we do not treat the disease at all.

How do we treat severe retinopathy of prematurity?

Currently, there are two options available for the treatment of severe ROP. The first one is laser surgery, also called "laser photocoagulation." The second is the intravitreal injection of an anti-VEGF agent such as Bevacizumab or Ranibizumab.

These two medications are also used in adults for the treatment of cancer. Their mechanism of action is such that they stop the development of new blood vessels in a tumor and starve it

DR WLODZIMIERZ M. WISNIEWSKI

of oxygen. The medications work similarly in babies. As you may remember, when I talked about aggressive forms of ROP, I explained that they are characterized by the fast growth of abnormal tortuous blood vessels. These two medications injected locally into the eyes are capable of stopping that abnormal growth in babies.

No large trials exist that would allow us to compare available treatment options. Both have advantages and disadvantages. It is good to have your baby treated in a center where both options are offered so that the best solution can be chosen. While deciding which treatment option to use, physicians and parents should take into account various factors. One of them is the *severity of the disease* and the doctor's experience and confidence with each technique. Laser therapy is a long-established therapy while anti-VEGF treatment is a newer technique, and we have less data on its efficacy and long-term visual and systemic outcomes. By systemic consequences, I mean potential effects on the baby's brain or other organs even though the medication is injected only locally into the baby's eyes.

The *timing of the response* after treatment will vary as well. ROP involution will most likely be faster after anti-VEGF therapy than after laser surgery. Finally, we should also consider the *burden for the baby*: can the baby tolerate the treatment well? Intravitreal administration of anti-VEGF agents can be done quickly and only with local topical anesthesia at the bedside. On the other hand, laser treatment will require much more time, will be more stressful for the baby, and will necessitate administration of general anesthesia.

Long-term vision outcomes may differ after each therapy. However, that has not been well documented yet. Later risk of myopia or shortsightedness appears to be lesser with anti-VEGF treatment. Some also speculate that anti-VEGF therapy might limit permanent peripheral visual field loss.

Prognosis and outcomes for premature babies with a diagnosis of retinopathy of prematurity

Children with a history of ROP (regardless of whether they required treatment or not) are at increased risk for the development of myopia (shortsightedness), astigmatism (distorted vision), and lazy eye. Therefore, they should be undergoing regular check-ups during childhood.

Data tells us that long-term visual impairment occurs in 7% to 15% of children with moderate to severe ROP. *The risk for an unfavorable visual outcome is highest for babies with ROP Stage 3 or higher and ROP in zone 1.*

ROP disease is often a more global indicator of severe complications that the baby was going through during their NICU stay. Severe ROP is a predictor of non-visual functional outcomes as well. In one study of 1,500 babies born with a birth weight below 1,250 g, it was found that 40% of babies with severe ROP had at least one non-visual disability compared with only 16% of babies without severe ROP. Motor developmental delays, cognitive impairments, and hearing loss were three to four times more likely to occur in children with a history of severe ROP than in children without it.

What questions to ask your neonatologist or eye-doctor if you have a premature baby in the neonatal intensive care unit?

1. Is my baby at risk for ROP?
2. If yes, when will the first ROP exam be done?

If your baby already has a ROP diagnosis, ask these questions:

1. How severe is ROP in my baby?
2. When will the next ROP exam be?
3. Does my baby need treatment for ROP, or are they likely to need treatment in the near future?

4. Do you provide both options (laser and medical) for the treatment of ROP in your hospital?
5. What is the long-term prognosis regarding my baby's vision?

Summary

I want to emphasize that ROP is a disease that affects most micro-preemies and extremely premature babies but not so much older preemies. Newborn babies are not born with this disease: they develop it over time during their hospitalization. The best approach to it, to prevent devastating outcomes such as loss of vision, is to be very vigilant. We have to start ROP screening exams at appropriate times and institute timely treatment when indicated. After discharge home, children who have had ROP will need regular follow-up to monitor their eye health.

CHAPTER 17

Intraventricular hemorrhage

I ntraventricular hemorrhage (IVH) is a brain injury that occurs mostly in premature babies and more frequently in the tiniest ones. It is crucial to know whether a baby has it, because it places babies at more risk for future developmental problems. As a neonatologist, I get many questions from parents of premature babies regarding this condition. I will explain here the risk factors, symptoms, diagnosis, and prognosis relating to IVH.

Basic information about intraventricular hemorrhage

Intraventricular hemorrhage – What is it?

If we cross-cut babies' brains, we will see solid areas called white and grey matter, and we will see fluid-filled chambers called ventricles. The role of the ventricles and the cerebrospinal fluid that fills them is to provide nutrition and protection for the brain tissue.

IVH is a condition in which blood vessels nourishing the brain rupture and blood gathers within the ventricles.

In mild IVH, blood is contained within the structure called the "germinal matrix," just near the wall of the ventricle. In more advanced bleeding, blood enters the ventricle and leads to its dilation.

Why does intraventricular hemorrhage occur in premature babies?

Doctors believe that premature babies are more prone to IVH due to increased fragility of blood vessels in the area of the germinal matrix, and also to unstable blood pressures in small premature babies. Premature babies after birth develop abnormal oxygen or carbon dioxide levels, unstable glucose levels, patent ductus arteriosus (PDA), metabolic imbalances, and anemia. These conditions may cause rapid changes in the blood flow and blood pressure within the brain, putting the baby at a higher risk of developing IVH.

Risk factors associated with an increased incidence of IVH are as follows:

- Lower gestational age at birth.
- Low Apgar scores and need for resuscitation after birth.
- Unstable blood pressures.
- Low oxygen levels.
- Abnormally low or high carbon dioxide levels.
- Severe anemia.
- Low platelets or clotting problems.
- Metabolic imbalances (abnormal levels of acid or glucose in the blood).

How common is intraventricular hemorrhage in premature babies?

Table 17.1: (Data adapted from Neonatal Outcomes of Extremely Preterm Infants from the NICHD Neonatal Research Network. Pediatrics. 2010 Sep; 126(3): 443–456.)

Gestational age at birth in weeks	23	24	25	26	27	28
IVH Grade 1+2	18%	21%	16%	12%	11%	8%
IVH Grade 3	15%	12%	8%	7%	6%	4%
IVH Grade 4	21%	14%	13%	7%	5%	3%

Intraventricular hemorrhage — clinical presentation

In most cases, an IVH occurs during the first day after birth, and almost all of them by the end of the first week of life. In 25% to 50% of cases, babies will have no obvious clinical symptoms, and IVH will be found only on a screening ultrasound study.

Symptoms of intraventricular hemorrhage

Babies who develop symptoms related to IVH may initially have subtle respiratory problems, an increased number of apneic episodes (pauses in breathing pattern), and muscle tone changes. In severe cases, we will witness seizures, flaccid muscle tone, severe apnea, stupor, and even coma.

How do we diagnose intraventricular hemorrhage?

The only way to diagnose IVH is by conducting brain imaging studies. The most common and the easiest is intracranial ultrasound. This is available in all hospitals and it can be done at the bedside without any special accommodations, even with the sickest newborn babies. The frequency and schedules for conducting ultrasounds will vary in different institutions. Most babies at risk will have one ultrasound during the first week of life, then at one month of age and the last study before discharge home.

If a baby has a positive ultrasound for IVH during the first week of life, we will continue doing ultrasounds weekly until it is determined that the baby is no longer at risk of developing any IVH complications.

Head CAT and magnetic resonance imaging (MRI) scans are more challenging to do on babies who are sick and being treated in a neonatal intensive care unit (NICU) on breathing machines. The significant advantage of CAT and MRI scans is that they allow us to obtain a better look into the baby's brain anatomy, and any damage that may have occurred there.

Based on radiographic appearance, we classify every IVH into a grade of 1 to 4.

Grade 1: bleeding that occurs within the germinal matrix adjacent to the ventricle.

Grade 2: bleeding that occupies up to 50% of the lateral ventricle volume.

Grade 3: bleeding that occupies more than 50% of the ventricle volume also causing ventricular dilation.

Grade 4: periventricular hemorrhage within the brain white matter coexistent with a significant lateral ventricular bleed on the same side.

Grades 1 and 2 are considered *mild bleeds*, and Grades 3 and 4 are *severe bleeds*.

Treatment of intraventricular hemorrhage in newborn babies

Sadly, there is no specific treatment for IVH. Management of a baby with diagnosed IVH will always include supportive therapy and constant surveillance for any complications.

Supportive therapy should include the following measures:

1. Correction of clotting problems and low platelet levels with appropriate transfusions.
2. Careful management of nutrition with emphasis on fluids, electrolytes, and glucose levels.
3. Ensuring adequate respiratory support to avoid low oxygen levels and abnormal carbon dioxide levels.
4. Control of blood flow and blood pressure to avoid hyper- and hypotension (abnormally high or low blood pressures).

5. Treatment of seizures with medications if indicated.
6. Continuous monitoring in the NICU on pulse-oximeters and cardiorespiratory monitors.

Serial monitoring of IVH with frequent cranial ultrasounds and measurements of the head circumference is essential. Some doctors will order ultrasound twice a week, and others will do them once a week. The goal is to follow the size of the ventricles, spot any obstruction in the flow of the cerebrospinal fluid, and look for hydrocephalus.

Sometimes, when ultrasound is not able to assess the degree of brain damage or aggressive intervention such as the placement of a ventriculoperitoneal (VP) shunt is needed, doctors may order a head CAT or MRI scan.

Complications and prognosis

Complications

Some babies, particularly those with IVH Grades 3 or 4, may progress to developing posthemorrhagic ventricular dilation (PHVD), also called "posthemorrhagic hydrocephalus." This complication is an important condition to watch for. PHVD may require therapeutic intervention and is associated with increased mortality and neurodevelopmental impairment during childhood. We suspect that PHVD is caused by an impaired ability to absorb cerebrospinal fluid due to inflammation after blood entered the ventricles.

Another type of ventricular dilation may occur due to the obstruction of cerebrospinal fluid flow caused by blood clots sitting within the ventricles.

PHVD is more common with more severe forms of IVH, at lower gestational ages, and when the baby is generally sicker. Usually, ventricular dilation begins 1 to 3 weeks after the onset of IVH. In up to 40% of cases, ventricular dilation stops progressing and does not need any intervention beyond close follow-up.

However, remaining cases will require treatment with frequent lumbar spinal taps or VP shunt placement.

VP shunt is a surgery used to treat hydrocephalus (severe dilation of the ventricles in the brain). During this procedure, a small flexible plastic tube is used, with one end placed in the ventricle and the other end in the peritoneal cavity (abdomen). Tubing will have a one-way valve that will allow drainage of cerebrospinal fluid out of the ventricles into the abdominal cavity. The idea is to decrease pressure on the brain and facilitate better growth of the brain tissue.

Prognosis

Different authors cite mortality rates of 20% to 30% for babies with Grade 3 IVH and 40% mortality rate for babies with IVH Grade 4. Authors of the study that summarized data from 1,812 babies who were born at fewer than 33 weeks of gestational age reported cerebral palsy rates for IVH Grades 1, 2, 3, and 4 being 8%, 11%, 19%, and 50%, respectively.[4]

It is still debatable whether infants with mild IVH (Grades 1 and 2) have a higher risk of neurodevelopmental impairment than survivors who do not have IVH.

Can we prevent intraventricular hemorrhage in premature babies?

There is no way to eliminate the occurrence of IVH. However, there are specific approaches believed to decrease its incidence and severity:

- Transporting mothers who are in premature labor at fewer than 32 weeks to level 3 centers.
- Treating mothers in early labor with steroids if indicated.

---

[4] Predictors of Cerebral Palsy in Very Preterm Infants: The EPIPAGE Prospective Population-Based Cohort Study. Dev Med Child Neurol, 2010 Jun; 52(6).

- Prompt treatment of amniotic sac infections (chorioamnionitis) with antibiotics.
- Treating mothers in premature labor with medications to slow down contractions and delay the birth of the baby.
- Timely and adequate resuscitation to avoid abnormal levels of oxygen and carbon dioxide.
- Avoiding giving fluid boluses but providing the appropriate treatment of low or high blood pressure.
- Avoidance of rapid changes in blood glucose or acid levels.
- Limiting the number of blood transfusions during the first few days of life.
- Treating clotting problems and low platelets levels if needed.
- Treatment of PDA (controversial as we still argue about the best approach to PDA)

What questions to ask if your baby suffers from intraventricular hemorrhage?

1. How do you grade the IVH that my baby has?
2. How often will you be doing brain imaging studies?
3. Does my baby have any complications from IVH?
4. What is the prognosis for the future neurodevelopment in my baby, given that they have IVH?

CHAPTER 18

Infections and use of antibiotics

Part 1. General Information

It is very common for premature babies to be placed on antibiotics at least once during their hospitalization. Many factors contribute to increased incidence of infections and frequent use of antibiotics among such babies in a neonatal intensive care unit (NICU).

Maternal infections may be one of the reasons leading to early labor and premature birth. Whenever a mother has fever, prolonged ruptured membranes, or infection of her amniotic sac, her baby will have a much higher chance of already being infected at birth. In addition to that, premature babies have an immature immunologic system and are more susceptible to various infections. Newborn babies receive antibodies that can fight infections from their mothers. However, that "gifting" of antibodies occurs mostly during the last 3 months, so premature babies don't get them in sufficient amounts. Finally, premature babies who stay in the NICU for several weeks or months are exposed to various procedures and therapies that increase the risk of infections. Being on a ventilator, or having intravenous (IV) catheters, tubes, and monitor leads on their body significantly increases a patient's chances of catching an infection.

Which microorganisms can affect newborn babies?

In the world of infectious diseases, the culprits are called "microorganisms." Bacteria, viruses, and yeasts are the three most important groups. I am not going to give you all their names, but I will mention the most common culprits here.

Bacterial infections, by far, are the most frequently diagnosed and treated infections in a NICU. If a mother suffers from syphilis, gonorrhea, chlamydia, or urinary tract infection, she can pass her microorganisms to the baby. Also, many mothers are carriers of Group B Streptococcus (GBS). This particular bacterium may cause severe infections in a baby, such as pneumonia, sepsis, or meningitis. Fortunately, GBS responds quickly to a common antibiotic—Penicillin. Babies who need a central line for a long time to receive IV nutrition are at risk of developing central line-associated bloodstream infection (CLABSI). The most common culprits of catheter-associated infections are Staphylococcus epidermidis and Staphylococcus aureus. Again, both are treatable with appropriate antibiotics.

Viruses are less of a problem for a newborn baby. However, when present, they are more challenging to treat because they do not respond as well as bacteria to antibiotics. They are also more likely to cause long-lasting consequences. Let's talk about three specific cases: Cytomegalovirus (CMV), Herpes, and respiratory illnesses.

CMV causes mild flu-like symptoms in adults and most of us do not even know that we have had this infection. However, if a pregnant woman acquires it, the fetus and, consequently, the future child may have long-lasting effects such as small head size, hearing deficits, vision deficits, calcifications in the brain, and lower intellectual potential.

Herpes virus, in adults, causes small ulcerative lesions in the mouth and genital area. The sores have a reddish rim surrounding them and are painful. Once Herpes is acquired, it never completely goes away: it becomes a recurrent infection whenever your immune system becomes weakened a little—for example, during pregnancy. Newborn babies can get infected whenever they come into contact with active lesions. That can occur during delivery (if the mother has genital Herpes) or after birth when the mother kisses her baby (if she has oral Herpes). Herpes can be a devastating disease for newborn babies. It can cause skin infections, pneumonia, infection of the central nervous system (encephalitis), and death. Despite antibiotic treatment, many survivors of Herpes infection will develop severe developmental impairment.

Respiratory viruses can affect premature babies during their stay in the NICU and beyond. Examples of such infections are influenza virus ('flu), respiratory syncytial virus (RSV), cold viruses, coronavirus, and many others. We may test for these viruses when we encounter unexplained deterioration in a baby's respiratory status. Unfortunately, we lack effective antibiotic treatments for them. RSV is the virus causing the most harm in premature babies and infants. Therefore, I describe it more thoroughly in Part 2 of this chapter.

Yeast infections affect babies because of their immature immune system and frequent exposure to antibiotics in the NICU that cause the eradication of "good bacteria" from their system. The most common fungal infection in babies is a diaper rash caused by Candida. This is relatively benign and easy to treat. More serious yeast infections occur when the microorganisms are found in blood or cerebrospinal fluid, or affect the heart or kidneys. The latter cases are much more challenging to treat and can lead to long-term adverse outcomes.

A special case—congenital infections

If a baby catches infection from their mother during pregnancy, this is called a "congenital infection." Except for two bacterial conditions (Syphilis and Listeria), most other congenital diseases are of viral or parasitic origin. Varicella (chickenpox), Herpes, CMV, Rubella, Parvovirus, Zika virus, and Toxoplasma are the microorganisms capable of causing congenital infections. Many affected babies will not have any symptoms at birth. Others will present with skin rashes, small head circumference, enlarged liver and spleen, abnormalities in the brain or eyes, or hearing deficits. It is better to prevent these conditions because the treatment of most of them will often not be beneficial. In many cases, congenital infections will negatively affect the baby's future development despite any treatment after birth. Before and during pregnancy, preventive measures should include avoidance of cats (Toxoplasma), getting all recommended vaccinations (Rubella, Varicella), and taking screening tests (Syphilis, Herpes).

Symptoms of infection and diagnostic process

Symptoms of infections in newborn babies are always non-specific. Any abnormality occurring in a newborn baby may be the first sign of infection. For example, feeding problems, increasing need for oxygen, more frequent apneas and temperature instability: all can be signs of an infection. That is why, whenever a baby has a new health problem, we always think first about infections and perform evaluations. We call these evaluations "screening for infection." We do these screenings often because late diagnosis and delay in treatment may have grave consequences for premature babies. As part of this process, we order tests using blood, urine, and spinal fluid. Depending on a particular situation, we may only use blood tests, blood, and urine, or all three. Sometimes we may also use other samples such as throat swabs, skin swabs, peritoneal fluids, or pus from an abscess. Whenever a baby has a positive blood culture (i.e. bacteria are growing in the blood), a lumbar puncture must be done, if not done before. Results from spinal fluid tests will determine the duration of necessary antibiotic treatment (e.g. 10 days versus 21 days).

Without getting too much into the diagnostic process, I want to divide all diagnostic tests into two groups. The first group comprises the tests that do not tell us whether an infection is present or not: they only change our level of suspicion. For example, abnormal urinalysis may be suggestive of urinary infection, or abnormal C-reactive protein may indicate a higher chance of sepsis (infection in the blood). We must also be aware of other conditions that can cause the same abnormalities but are not infectious diseases.

The second group of tests lets us know whether an infection is present and gives the culprit's name. All types of cultures, DNA probes, and polymerase chain reaction (PCR) tests belong in this group. Unfortunately, these tests are sometimes not 100% accurate (they miss actual infection) and the results may take even several days to come back. That is the reason why we start treatment with antibiotics whenever we "just" suspect an infection. Furthermore, sometimes, even when culture study is negative but the patient improved after antibiotics had been started, we might decide to finish the full course of treatment rather than stopping antibiotics too early.

Approach to treatment

Most bacterial infections are treatable if antibiotics are started early. Occasionally, there will be bacteria that are difficult to treat because of their resistance to antibiotics. The treatment duration will vary from 1 to 2 weeks for urinary, lung, and blood infections, 2 to 3 weeks for meningitis, and several weeks to several months for bone infections (osteomyelitis).

Treating viral infections is always very difficult because we have medications only against a few viruses and the medicines are not very effective.

The treatment of yeast infections is also prolonged. It usually takes a much longer time to eradicate fungus from our system than bacteria. It is not uncommon for a baby to need anti-fungal medication for several weeks before the infection can be cleared entirely.

In most severe cases of infection, newborn babies may need to be placed on a ventilator, and receive IV fluids and medications to support their blood pressure. We need to be vigilant in recognizing any disturbance in vital organs and supporting their functions as required.

What is the prognosis if your baby gets an infection in the neonatal intensive care unit?

We doctors take all infections very seriously because one can die of them. Fortunately, many infections are treatable with antibiotics if recognized early. We have many excellent medicines available for bacterial and yeast infections. However, therapeutic agents against viruses are not very effective.

Prognosis regarding survival is more guarded in patients with unstable blood pressure or requiring placement on a ventilator. Neurodevelopmental outcomes are more likely to be poor in patients in whom infection attacked the central nervous system (meningitis or encephalitis). One should remember, though, that statistics are just that: numbers. Even among babies who have had meningitis and severe sepsis with unstable blood pressures, there will be children with normal developmental outcomes.

Part 2. Respiratory syncytial virus (RSV) in premature babies and infants

RSV is a virus that attacks the respiratory system, specifically the upper and lower airways. It may affect your child in the NICU or after discharge home. One can contract RSV infection by inhaling droplets from the air if you are in the proximity of a sick patient, or by direct contact with viruses—for example, by touching contaminated surfaces and transferring those secretions to your nasal cavity or your eyes. RSV affects people of all ages but is most dangerous to infants, especially former micro-preemies and very premature babies. In those babies, it is more likely to lead to severe apnea and pneumonia. (Apnea is defined as a pause in breathing; pneumonia is an infection of the lungs.)

It is worth mentioning that up to 3% of all infants under a year old may need hospitalization due to lower respiratory tract infection caused by RSV. Fortunately, most babies who were previously healthy do well and stay in the hospital for no more than 2 to 3 days. Sadly, in the USA, about 100 babies per year will have died each year due to this disease. The infection is so common that, by 24 months of age, almost all children have had it at least once.

When sick, pretty much all affected pediatric patients will have decreased activity, poor appetite, or difficulties with feeding. They will also have a runny nose with a lot of secretions and low-grade fever. In infants with involvement of the lower respiratory airways, we will often see nasal flaring, grunting (making noise while exhaling air), retractions, and need for additional oxygen while breathing. These latter symptoms can also be described as "increased work of breathing." It occurs due to airways getting plugged by secretions. Secretions lead to increased resistance in the airways, making babies work harder when trying to inhale and exhale air.

How do we diagnose respiratory syncytial virus infection?

The diagnosis of RSV is relatively straightforward. If we get a pediatric patient, especially an infant presenting with respiratory symptoms without a previous diagnosis of asthma during the RSV season (October—March), we should suspect RSV infection. To confirm the diagnosis, we can do a nasal swab for secretions and perform so-called "rapid testing" or send the sample for RSV culture. The rapid test will yield results within an hour. RSV culture will take several days to come back. In most cases, confirming RSV infection is not that crucial since we do not have specific treatments for it. More important is to rule out other more dangerous conditions—for example, bacterial infections. If bacterial infections are not recognized quickly, they can lead to sepsis (overwhelming infection of the whole body) and even death.

How do we treat respiratory syncytial virus infections?

There is no specific treatment for RSV infections. The treatment is supportive. What does that mean? We will be supporting patients' symptoms, trying to alleviate their severity.

For fever, we will give anti-fever medications. If a baby is unable to eat because of poor appetite or nasal secretions, we can provide milk using a nasogastric tube or start IV fluids. If the baby has consistently low oxygen levels, we can provide supplementary oxygen for breathing. If the baby has copious nasal secretions, we will suction them frequently to ease breathing effort. In rare situations, for patients with severely compromised respiratory function, we will use a ventilator.

The following medications are not helpful in routine treatment of RSV infections:

- Albuterol treatment.
- Steroids.
- Nebulized epinephrine.
- Ribavirin.
- RSV immunoglobulins as a treatment.
- Routine antibiotics without evidence of bacterial infection.

Can we prevent respiratory syncytial virus infections?

We can prevent RSV infections by eliminating or minimizing exposure to the virus. We can also decrease the severity of the infection by giving RSV immunoglobulin to the most vulnerable individuals. Remember, adults and older children can get RSV infection and can infect others. Decreasing exposure occurs by making sure that we frequently wash our hands. We must always wash hands before and after encountering a new environment such as a new room, a church, a shop, or a person, particularly a sick person. Also, extremely important is that we avoid touching our faces with our hands. Introducing infectious viruses to our mucous membranes in eyes, nose, and mouth significantly increases the chances of getting sick.

Vulnerable infants such as babies who were born very prematurely, or ones who suffer from certain congenital heart conditions or chronic lung diseases, can be protected to a certain degree with RSV immunoglobulin. RSV immunoglobulin called Palivizumab is an antibody produced using DNA technology. It prevents the virus from entering human cells and slows down its multiplication and proliferation. Palivizumab is believed to reduce the risks of RSV affecting the lower respiratory tract. It may also decrease the number of hospital admissions due to the disease. So far, we do not have any proof that the medication reduces RSV-related mortality or subsequent childhood asthma. We still debate how useful and cost-effective RSV immunoglobulin is. Therefore, recommendations for this medication's administration keep changing.

Health insurance companies and professional organizations have developed various recommendations regarding which patients should be treated with RSV immunoglobulin, when, and how many times. If an infant qualifies for therapy with Palivizumab, the treatment should be started at the beginning of the RSV season. The medication should be given once a month as an intramuscular injection and for no more than five doses. In cases where the baby acquires infection and is admitted to the hospital, prophylaxis can be stopped.

The following infants may be given RSV prophylaxis:

1. Preterm infants born at fewer than 29 weeks of gestation and who are younger than 1 year at the start of the RSV season.
2. Preterm infants born at fewer than 32 weeks of gestation who developed the need for oxygen for more than 28 days and who are younger than 1 year at the start of the RSV season.

3. Babies who were born at fewer than 32 weeks and are still treated for chronic lung disease with medications or oxygen and are younger than 2 years at the start of the RSV season.
4. Children with congenital heart conditions after cardiology consultation to check whether they are likely to benefit from the prevention.

But note that a diagnosis of either Down syndrome or cystic fibrosis by itself is not an indication for the RSV prophylaxis.

(I have only listed some indications for RSV prophylaxis in infants. For a full list of recommendations, refer to the Centers for Disease Control and Prevention (CDC) guidelines, the American Academy of Pediatrics (AAP) guidelines, Red Book, and your health insurance organization. Remember that these recommendations tend to change very often.)

Are there any long-term consequences after RSV infections?

Most patients affected by RSV infections recover without any long-term negative outcomes. However, there is some data to suggest that infants who had infections of the lower respiratory airways, such as pneumonia or bronchiolitis, during the first months of life are prone to developing wheezing episodes later on in their lives.

CHAPTER 19

Anemias and blood products transfusions

B lood consists of two major components: cells and liquid. Red blood cells (RBCs), white blood cells (leukocytes), and platelets constitute the cellular part. RBCs carry oxygen to tissues, white cells defend us from infections, and platelets are responsible for clotting or preventing bleeding. The liquid portion is called "plasma" or "serum." It consists of water and numerous chemical compounds needed in our body such as proteins, fat, sugars, antibodies against infections, and clotting factors.

Depending on a specific condition, virtually any component of the blood may be in an insufficient amount, an excessive amount, or, despite normal levels, malfunctioning.

I do not want this chapter to become a textbook on hematology, so, in Part 1, I will only concentrate on the most common blood-related condition occurring in premature babies called "anemia." In Part 2, I will discuss transfusions of different blood products that may be necessary for patients in a neonatal intensive care unit (NICU).

Anemia is defined by an abnormally low number of RBCs. However, we can also use other measures, such as hemoglobin or hematocrit, to help us with the diagnosis. Hemoglobin is a protein in the RBCs that is responsible for attaching to and carrying oxygen. Therefore, hemoglobin is an indirect indicator of the number of RBCs. The average hemoglobin value in a newborn is 15–16 gm/dl. Hematocrit is a ratio of RBC volume to total blood volume, and the average value in a neonate is around 55%.

Part 1. Anemia

There are literally hundreds of causes for anemia in a baby. I will talk briefly about the three most common situations that can occur in the NICU.

1. *Blood loss during pregnancy and labor*. If anemia is present right after birth, it is most likely due to acute or chronic blood loss experienced by the baby as a result of placental abruption, placenta previa, or feto-maternal bleeding (the baby is "donating" its blood to the mother). Affected babies may need an emergency transfusion of packed red blood cells (PRBCs) immediately after birth (usually, we transfuse PRBCs instead of the whole blood).
2. *Blood loss due to testing*. After admitting a baby to the NICU, doctors will order numerous blood tests: the sicker the baby is, the more tests will be done. In the end, all blood tests add up to a significant amount of blood loss and cause anemia. You should know that baby has only about 80 ml of blood for each kilogram of body weight (1kg = 2.2 lb). The tiniest babies are the ones who are most affected. Due to the severity of their condition, they need frequent blood tests while, at the same time, their total blood volume is very low.
3. *Blood groups incompatibility* between the mother and the baby may cause anemia in babies. When the mother has blood type "O" in the ABO system or "Rh-negative" in the RH system, she may pass antibodies to the baby that will react with the baby's red cells. The reaction is called

"hemolysis" and it may result in anemia, but only if the baby's blood type is A, B, or Rh-positive. In addition to anemia, this situation may also lead to more severe jaundice (jaundice = yellow skin; see Chapter 10).

The treatment of neonatal anemia involves minimizing further blood loss, providing proper nutrition containing iron and folic acid, and blood transfusions. Some centers also utilize subcutaneous erythropoietin injections. Erythropoietin is a natural hormone capable of stimulating bone marrow to produce red cells. However, it works slowly (taking 2 to 4 weeks to see a response), and there are differing opinions on its utility in the NICU.

Part 2. Blood products in the neonatal intensive care unit

Each component of the blood has its specific function. Therefore, we try to transfuse only the ones that are needed and most likely to benefit the baby. We always balance risks and benefits and do not make decisions to transfuse blood products lightly.

Transfusion of packed red blood cells (PRBC)

This is the most commonly performed transfusion in the NICU. When your doctor tells you that they want to transfuse blood to your baby, it usually means PRBC transfusion. When a patient has anemia, we do not want to transfuse whole blood. Instead, we transfuse concentrated RBCs without other cellular components and excess of a liquid part. There is considerable variability in the criteria for blood transfusion. Doctors will consider it in a baby on a ventilator who is requiring a large amount of oxygen and has a hematocrit of 30% to 40%. A hematocrit of around 20% will be an indication in a stable patient with chronic anemia who does not respond to iron and nutritional treatments. As you can see from my examples, for sicker patients who need oxygen, we have more liberal criteria for blood transfusion (remember: RBCs carry oxygen to our tissues).

Platelet transfusions

Generally, newborns should have more than 150,000/cubic millimeter of platelets. Depending on the actual number and other factors, indications to have platelet transfusion will differ. Again, a reminder: platelets protect us from bleeding. Premature babies are naturally at risk of having bleeding in the brain or blood loss post-surgery. Most surgeons would request a pre-surgery platelet transfusion if the baby's platelets were below 80,000. In a stable "older" premature baby without brain bleed, we may delay transfusion until the platelets drop below 30,000 to 50,000. During the procedure, we transfuse only platelet mass without a significant amount of other blood components.

Fresh frozen plasma transfusion

Plasma contains numerous non-cellular clotting factors. Therefore, fresh frozen plasma (FFP) transfusion is indicated after major surgeries when there is a high risk of bleeding or in severely sick premature babies with necrotizing enterocolitis (NEC) (see Chapter 13).

Double volume exchange blood transfusion

During this procedure, we remove the baby's blood from its body and replace it with blood from a blood bank. The main indication is uncontrolled hyperbilirubinemia (yellow skin) endangering future brain function (more details in Chapters 10 and 20).

What are the potential complications after blood products transfusions?

Occasionally, blood transfusions may cause complications. Blood may be a source of allergic reactions, infections, metabolic abnormalities, exaggerated immune responses, and post-transfusion NEC. Although blood donors and all donated blood are extensively tested, there is always a small risk for problems. NICU staff always pay extreme attention to ensuring that each baby receives the "right" unit of blood (correctly matched, tested, and labeled). Most NICUs have a policy that two nurses or a nurse with a doctor have to check blood labeling independently before it can be processed and given to a baby. Administration of the blood products takes several hours, during which we monitor your baby very carefully. We will be checking more frequently their temperature, heart rate, respiratory rate, and blood pressure. If, based on those observations, we suspect any serious adverse reaction to the blood products, we will stop transfusion immediately.

Can a father or a family member donate blood for a baby?

Sometimes, parents or family members want to donate and dedicate a unit of blood to their child. Although not impossible, this is often impractical. First of all, it is a misconception that blood donated by family members is safer than the blood from the blood bank. Anybody, including the patient's family members, goes through the same screening procedures before being allowed to donate blood. In addition, a baby often needs transfusion urgently but arranging for the family to donate blood will take more time. It is preferable that family members give blood to the blood bank, but into a general pool, because blood is a very precious resource and we never have too much of it. If you feel strongly and prefer to donate blood only for your child, talk about it ahead of time, preferably right after the admission of your baby to the NICU.

CHAPTER 20

Diagnostic and therapeutic procedures

E ach medical specialty has some specific procedures. Certain approaches are unique to neonatal care, and others are similar to those used in other medical fields. In this chapter, I want to give you an overview of the standard procedures encountered in the neonatal intensive care unit (NICU). My goal is to familiarize you with them, not to give you a full description of how the procedure is performed. I will mention some indications, benefits, and complications associated with these interventions, but my list will not be complete. You need to ask relevant questions when you talk with your baby's doctor before giving your consent to anything. Certain procedures may be done without your written permission because they will be considered emergent and, if done soon after birth, you might still be recovering from the anesthesia and we would not be able to talk to you.

Cardiorespiratory resuscitation (reviving or "stabilizing" your baby)

Many tiny babies after birth require reviving measures. Whenever we have to support their breathing effort or heart function, we say that we conducted cardiorespiratory resuscitation (CPR). CPR includes several steps:

1. Drying, warming the baby, and suctioning secretions from the mouth and nose with a concurrent evaluation of respiratory effort and heart rate.
2. Provision of external breaths for a baby who is not breathing or breathing inadequately. We do this by using a bag connected to a mask placed on the baby's face or a bag attached to a breathing tube placed in the baby's windpipe. By squeezing the bag, we are pushing air with extra oxygen into the baby's lungs. If the baby needs artificial breaths (external breaths) for a longer time, we will connect them to a ventilator, usually in the NICU.
3. Chest compressions - If, despite providing external breaths, the baby has a low or absent heart rate, we will start chest compressions. We do this by placing our fingers above the heart. Chest compressions in effect are squeezing the heart and circulating blood in the baby's body. If the baby still does not respond despite all previous measures, we insert an umbilical venous catheter (UVC, see below) and use this to administer medications and fluids.

Fluid administration and blood draws

Premature babies born at fewer than 32 weeks always require intravenous (IV) fluids and blood draws for testing. The chances are that your baby will need at least one of the below-described procedures.

Umbilical venous catheter (UVC)

After the birth, the umbilical cord is cut and clamped, so blood does not ooze out from it. There are three large vessels in an umbilical cord: two arteries and one vein (rare exceptions exist). UVC access can be used during resuscitation or after birth when the baby is small, and we consider peripheral IV access to be suboptimal. We use a catheter: a thin, flexible, plastic tube that we gently insert into the umbilical vein and advance to a pre-determined depth, hoping to position its tip in a large vessel close to the heart. Sometimes, the catheter goes into the liver or other areas where it cannot be left safely. UVC placement can be done quickly at the bedside or during resuscitation. It requires an x-ray to confirm the proper position of the catheter tip. Once in place, we can use the UVC for several days. It is used mainly for the administration of fluids, IV nutrition, and medications. Occasionally, we can also draw blood from it.

Umbilical arterial catheter (UAC)

This is placed in patients in whom we expect the frequent need for blood tests and want to monitor blood pressure continuously. We perform this procedure soon after birth, usually at the same time as we place a UVC. The catheter is placed in an umbilical artery and advanced to the desired position. An x-ray will be required to confirm the safe location of the catheter tip. Sometimes, babies develop adverse reactions to this catheter. One of the arteries may vaso-constrict, causing a change in the color of the foot or leg. If you ever notice bluish, greyish, or pale discoloration of one extremity in your baby who has a UAC, notify their nurse immediately.

Radial artery catheter

Radial artery is a vessel located in the area of the wrist in both our hands. We can insert a radial catheter in older newborns to monitor blood pressure and for frequent blood draws. We do

not place it in tiny babies because the radial artery might be too small. Right after birth, we prefer to obtain a UAC rather than a radial artery catheter because UAC placement is easier. Beyond seven days after delivery, though, a UAC is not an option because the umbilicus will be dry and it becomes too difficult to place any umbilical catheters. The radial catheter may sometimes compromise adequate blood flow to the hand. Therefore, if you notice the hand's discoloration, notify your nurse immediately.

Peripherally inserted central catheter (PICC)

This is a central IV access. Both UVCs and PICCs are IV lines providing central access, which means that the catheter tip will be located in a larger vessel close to the heart. Using central lines, we can offer the most optimal IV nutrition to the baby (i.e. a higher concentration of sugar, protein, and fat). For the PICC, we use an extremely thin and flexible plastic catheter. After thoroughly cleaning the skin, we use a needle introducer to puncture a small vein on a hand or leg, and then we try to thread a catheter into it and advance it to the desired length. As with other catheter placements, we need to obtain an x-ray to confirm the catheter tip's correct location.

Simple peripheral IV access

We can place a short plastic catheter in peripheral veins, usually on hands, feet, or elbow areas. Peripheral IV access is not a preferable option to deliver fluids and medications to a tiny baby after birth. It is difficult to place and may be lost easily, necessitating repeat procedures. Most babies who need IV access for longer than seven days will require a UVC or PICC.

Hill stick (or "hill prick")

This is a frequent procedure in a NICU. We use it to obtain a small amount of blood for testing. A nurse will clean the hill area (on a foot), prick it with a small lancet, and drip drops of blood into a container by gently squeezing the foot. Once the procedure is finished, she will wipe off the remainder of the blood and place a band-aid.

Respiratory system

Endotracheal intubation and placement on a ventilator

The procedure during which we place a breathing tube (endotracheal tube = ET-tube) into a baby's windpipe is called "endotracheal intubation." We perform it during prolonged CPR in the delivery room or in the NICU when we expect that the baby will need a ventilator or treatment with surfactant. To do that, we use the plastic tube with a diameter of 2 to 3.5 mm and place it between the vocal cords into the windpipe. It is a somewhat tricky procedure and, in most cases, requires an x-ray to confirm that the tip of the ET-tube is in the right place. Having an ET-tube in place allows us to provide external breaths more efficiently.

Surfactant administration

Surfactant is a specific medication that we use to treat moderate and severe respiratory distress syndrome (see Chapter 8). It is a liquid milky substance that we instill directly into a baby's lungs using an ET-tube. If the baby is already on a ventilator, it will have the ET-tube in place; otherwise, we will perform endotracheal intubation first. In most cases, the surfactant will improve lung function and decrease the need for oxygen quite rapidly.

Chest tube placement

A ruptured lung, also called a "pneumothorax," is a severe complication occurring in some babies with respiratory problems. A small portion of the lung may rupture, air leaks out and gathers between the chest wall and the lung, preventing lung expansion. Placement of a needle or chest tube in the chest cavity to evacuate the air may become necessary. Once a chest tube is placed, it is usually left in for several hours or days. Sometimes we just use the needle first, as a one-time procedure to diagnose the condition and treat it. However, if one attempt at needling is not curative, chest tube placement may be necessary. In most cases, the procedure is urgent. We would perform it at the bedside after using a local anesthetic. We make a small cut in the skin on the chest, spread some tissues with instruments, and place a plastic tube directly into the chest cavity. Once the tube is secured, we would connect it to a suction machine to keep evacuating any unnecessary air. As with other procedures, an x-ray is necessary to evaluate the tube's position and lung expansion.

Digestive system

Nasogastric or orogastric tube placement

All babies born at fewer than 32 weeks will have feeding problems. Newborns start acquiring proper coordination of sucking, swallowing, and breathing only around 32 to 34 weeks of gestational age. Hence, most very premature babies need tube feedings. We can place a small plastic tube through the nose (an NG-tube) or mouth (an OG-tube) down into the stomach and leave it there for many days to serve as a tool to provide milk. Many babies will need that tube until they reach 37 or even 42 weeks of corrected gestational age. For the minority of babies who never learn how to eat by mouth, surgeons can place a special apparatus on the baby's abdomen (a gastrostomy tube, or "G-tube"), which serves the same purpose.

Abdominal paracentesis

"Abdominal paracentesis" is a name for a procedure during which we insert a needle into the abdominal cavity to aspirate the excess of fluid or blood. In most cases, a surgeon would do this at the bedside but there are rare circumstances when it could be needed urgently during resuscitation, and then a neonatologist should be able to do it. The procedure may be required in tiny babies who develop complications of necrotizing enterocolitis in severe abdominal infections or rare congenital anomalies.

Urinary system

Whenever we suspect an infection in a baby older than a few days, we need to consider testing urine for urinary tract infections. To do this, we need a clean, uncontaminated urine sample. We can obtain urine for various studies by inserting a urine catheter through the urethra (= bladder catheterization). However, sometimes this procedure is complicated due to the small size of the urethra, or it does not yield any urine. Then we can try performing a "suprapubic urine collection." After the proper cleaning, we can insert a small needle in the lower abdomen. The needle will get into the bladder, and we can aspirate residing urine there for the necessary tests. If the urinary bladder is full, the procedure is relatively easy and does not require any x-rays.

Cardiovascular system

ECG

An ECG is a study allowing us to look at the heart's rhythm and the electric function of the heart. We order it when a baby has a low, high, or irregular heart rate. We will also do it if the baby has any congenital heart disease diagnosed on an "echo."

Echo

An "echo" is an ultrasound study enabling the visualization of the heart's anatomy to ensure that all structures are developed and aligned correctly. We order an echo in babies if we hear a heart murmur or suspect that a baby's health problems may be due to congenital heart disease.

Holter monitoring

Holter monitoring is a study similar to an ECG but conducted over an extended period, such as 12 to 24 hours. We will use a Holter monitor if a baby is known to have irregular heartbeats, and we want to determine their frequency and severity.

Electric shock therapy for the heart (cardioversion or defibrillation)

In rare situations, when a baby has severe heart arrhythmia leading to significant compromise of vital organ functions, electric shock therapy may be needed. This is applied by placing two electrodes on the baby's upper body and providing a single electric shock. Usually, a cardiologist (heart specialist) will be involved in making decisions about this therapy because, whenever feasible, we prefer trying medicinal solutions first.

Pericardiocentesis

The heart is located in a sac called the "pericardium." There are rare situations when we have to stick a needle in this sac to evacuate infectious fluid, IV fluid (if complications arise from the central catheter), blood, or free air. The procedure is called "pericardiocentesis." A cardiologist or neonatologist can perform the procedure and, if it is not urgent, they will use ultrasound to help direct the needle correctly.

Central nervous system

Lumbar or spinal tap

A lumbar tap (also called a "spinal tap") is a procedure during which we collect spinal fluid for various studies. A spinal tap may be necessary when we suspect an infection or congenital hormonal, metabolic, or genetic diseases. We also do it in babies with hydrocephalus: it is a therapeutic procedure in this case (see Chapter 17 about intraventricular hemorrhage [IVH]). For the procedure, we place the baby either in a sitting or side-lying position, bend its back, and insert a needle in the lumbar area. If you had spinal anesthesia for your delivery, it is a similar procedure to that, except that we don't inject anything into the baby.

Electroencephalogram

An electroencephalogram (EEG) is a study of electrical brain activity. We obtain it by placing multiple electrodes on a baby's head and recording results using the EEG machine. The most common indication for an EEG is when we suspect seizures in a baby. Also, if we want to declare a patient to be "brain dead," we might use this technique together with other methods.

Head ultrasound

Head ultrasound is the most commonly used brain imaging study in a NICU. We use it to screen babies for IVH, a brain bleed that may occur in some very premature babies. The head ultrasound is easy to do: it can be done at the bedside and is non-invasive.

Head CAT and MRI scans

CAT and MRI scans of the head can provide us with much more detail regarding brain anatomy than a head ultrasound. Unfortunately, they take more time and, with rare exception, the baby has to be transported to the radiology department to have it done. Congenital brain abnormalities, metabolic diseases, severe IVH, or hydrocephalus will be indications to do these studies.

A ventriculoperitoneal shunt

A ventriculoperitoneal (VP) shunt placement is a therapeutic procedure performed in babies with severe and progressive hydrocephalus (see Chapter 17 on IVH). Neurosurgeons do it. During the surgery, the doctor places one end of the catheter in the brain area called the "ventricle," then threads it under the skin and puts the other end in the abdominal cavity. The catheter will allow for a one-directional flow of the fluid if the pressure of the liquid in the brain exceeds a certain level. The goal is to relieve the pressure on the brain caused by excessive amounts of the fluid in the ventricles (hydrocephalus is defined as "enlargement of the ventricles in the brain").

Blood products

Transfusions

Premature babies may need transfusions of several blood products: red blood cells, platelets, or plasma. I explained more about transfusions in Chapter 19, so I will only emphasize here that the blood products typically come from a blood bank. They are tested for compatibility and are sterile.

Exchange transfusion

Exchange transfusion, or "double volume blood exchange transfusion," is a procedure used to treat very severe newborn jaundice that does not respond well to phototherapy (see Chapter 10). To perform exchange transfusion, we have to arrange for a large volume of blood from the blood bank, and we must ensure that the type of blood is appropriate for the patient. Then, we place a catheter (UVC) and use it to sequentially draw blood out of the baby's circulation and then replace it with the blood from the blood bank. We repeat this sequence many times, using small aliquots of blood to not overwhelm the heart with rapidly changing blood volumes.

CHAPTER 21

Outcomes of premature babies

Outcomes of premature babies are always on parents' minds. Parents want to know whether their baby will live, what kind of problems and complications they will endure in the neonatal intensive care unit (NICU), and what their quality of life will be after discharge home. In this chapter, I will provide you with some answers to these important questions.

Reading about the chance that your baby may not survive or will be at risk of having developmental problems in the future may be very upsetting. Do not proceed any further if you are a person who would rather not know the complete picture and if it is going to make you uncomfortable or sad.

Before I get into details and numbers, let me give you some advice on interpreting statistics. Whenever possible, I will provide you with data that have come from a large group of patients, say hundreds or thousands. This means that the numbers will be a function of both mildly sick patients and severely ill ones. Your baby is just one patient and, depending on their particular situation, the rate of survival or rate of complications will be either higher than cited or lower. Additionally, it always matters whether numerical results were gathered from patients similar to your child: for example, in the same healthcare system and comparably developed country. If you live in Venezuela with a poorly designed healthcare infrastructure, and the data I quoted came from Sweden or Canada, your child's outcomes may be much worse than those I cited. Finally, even if your child's probability of survival and normal motor and intellectual development is very low, it does not mean that your baby cannot be an exception. I can assure you: I have seen at least several gravely ill infants during my career who surprised me when they survived and later had a healthy normal childhood.

If your child is receiving treatment in a large neonatal center, the best source of statistics will be your neonatologist. All NICUs providing care to premature babies diligently gather statistical data on survival and complication rates in their patients. The purpose is to ensure that we are providing an excellent quality of care to all our patients and finding opportunities for improvement. There are two potential problems with this approach. First, data is not usually audited and publicly available. Second, unless statistics come from many patients (in my opinion, at least 100 babies similar to yours), such data is not very meaningful.

We can divide all neonatal outcomes into two groups: short term (occurring in the NICU) and long term (occurring after discharge home). Most of the medical conditions I have explained so far in this book belong to short-term outcomes. Problems such as temperature instability, poor feedings, respiratory issues including apneas, and jaundice afflict almost all newborns in a NICU who were born before 32 weeks. On the other hand, certain complications affect only some patients. Not all babies develop bronchopulmonary dysplasia (BPD), retinopathy of prematurity (ROP), necrotizing enterocolitis (NEC), intraventricular hemorrhage (IVH), or late infections. The general rule for the incidence of these severe complications is that the more premature and smaller babies have more of them. I have already written separate chapters on BPD, ROP, NEC,

IVH, and infections. Here, I want to concentrate on neonatal survival rates and long-term motor and intellectual outcomes.

Will my baby survive?

If I have enough forewarning before premature delivery occurs, I go to parents to have a conversation about the birth and their future child. If not, our first talk takes place after I have admitted the baby to the NICU and provided initial stabilization. Invariably, parents ask me the question, "Is our baby going to be OK?" What they mean is whether their baby will survive and how they will do in the future. So, let's first talk about survival rates for various gestational ages and the limits of viability.

Every year in the USA, more than 5,000 babies with a weight of fewer than 500 g (1.1 lb) are born, so the question, "What is the threshold of viability" is crucial to answer. Citing from *Williams Obstetrics*, 25th edition, "the threshold of viability lies between 20 and 26 weeks." You may ask why a given range of dates is so broad (six weeks). It is impossible to assign one date or one gestational week, after which the baby will have a chance to survive. Each of us human beings is very different in appearance and health. One is very tall, another short; one is obese and another slim; one is very healthy, and another is getting sick all the time. The same rule applies to newborn babies. Some babies are more mature at the same gestational age than others, and female newborns are usually more mature than boys. Also, white and Asian babies have better survival rates for the same gestational age and weight than black babies. Ultimately, parents with the help of neonatologists and obstetricians will have to decide whether to offer cardiopulmonary resuscitation (CPR) and treatment to their child, and under what circumstances to stop it. These are the most difficult decisions for all of us. As doctors, we understand that families will make different decisions under the same circumstances. Their choices will be influenced by personal experiences, religious beliefs, and understanding of data presented to them by doctors. If it is technologically feasible, we will almost always abide by parents' wishes.

Information on survival rates and developmental outcomes is crucial to the families' decision-making process, so let's talk about it now.

In 2017 (in the USA), 67% of all infant deaths occurred in newborns born preterm at fewer than 37 weeks of gestational age. Below, I present mortality rates per 1,000 live births by gestational age at birth (data from the Centers for Disease Control and Prevention, a US governmental agency):

- >42 weeks = 3.98 deaths per 1,000 live births;
- 37–41 weeks = 2.1 deaths per 1,000 live births;
- 34–36 weeks = 8.5 deaths per 1,000 live births;
- 32–33 weeks = 20.5 deaths per 1,000 live births;
- <32 weeks = 187.5 deaths per 1,000 live births.

Gestational age at birth is a particularly strong factor influencing babies' outcomes for the group of babies born before 32 weeks. Let's look at survival rates for those babies reported in two separate studies.

Rysavy, with his colleagues, published an article in the *New England Journal* in 2015, where he presented statistics from 24 large US hospitals, many being university centers.[5] The data covers information on almost 5,000 babies born before 27 weeks between 2006 and 2011. Survival rates are given in percentages for each gestational age from 22 to 26 weeks, provided doctors chose to offer active treatment. In brackets, I have included survival rates for babies born at 22 and 23 weeks regardless of whether active treatment was provided. This is a cause for a significant difference. Per parental wishes, the authors only offered aggressive treatment to 5% to 30% of babies born at 22 weeks,

---

5   Between-Hospital Variation in Treatment and Outcomes in Extreme Preterm Infants. Mathew A Rysavy et al. New England Journal of Medicine May 2015. https://www.nejm.org/doi/full/10.1056/nejmoa1410689

and 50% to 75% of babies born at 23 weeks of gestational age. Because including all babies for the calculation of survival rates increases the denominator only, the numbers in brackets are lower. Starting from 24 weeks, the vast majority of babies received comprehensive treatment. Therefore, I have reported only single values for respective gestational ages (GAs):

- 22 weeks of GA = 23% (5.1%) survival rate;
- 23 weeks of GA = 33% (23.6%) survival rate;
- 24 weeks of GA = 56.6% survival rate;
- 25 weeks of GA = 72% survival rate;
- 26 weeks of GA = 81% survival rate.

In 2017, Veronique Pierrat published the second dataset I want to present to you.[6] This article covers approximately 5,000 births before 35 weeks that occurred in France during 2011. Note that the authors broke down gestational ages differently from the previous report: they used ranges rather than single weeks, and they included babies until 34 weeks of gestational age. Reported survival rates represent survival data obtained at about two years after birth.

- 22–23 weeks of GA = 0% survival;
- 24 weeks = 29.2% survival rate;
- 25–26 weeks of GA = 66.6% survival rate;
- 27–31 weeks of GA = 94% survival rate;
- 32–34 weeks of GA = 97.7% survival rate.

As you can see, the survival rates for the tiniest babies in France were much lower than for those in the USA. The difference

---

[6] Neurodevelopmental Outcome at 2 Years for Preterm Children Born at 22–34 Weeks' Gestation in France in 2011: EPIPAGE-2 Cohort study. Veronique Pierrat et al. BMJ 2017. https://www.bmj.com/content/358/bmj.j3448#:~:text=Only%20one%20infant%20born%20at%20 22%2D23%20weeks%20survived.&text=Conclusions%20In%20this%20 large%20cohort,high%20risk%20of%20developmental%20delay

can be explained by a different approach to treating these babies in the two countries. The authors of the French study reported that in 2011 intensive care would have been withheld or withdrawn for 92% of babies born at 22 to 23 weeks of gestational age, whereas, as I mentioned above, up to 30% of babies at 22 weeks and 75% at 23 weeks of gestational age had received reviving treatments in the USA.

How is my baby going to do in the future?

The second frequently asked question on outcomes is about the quality of life and the possibility that the baby may have disabilities after discharge home. Disability is defined as "a physical or mental impairment that significantly limits one's life activities." It could be cerebral palsy, blindness, deafness, speech impairment, or lower intellectual potential. Often, one child may be affected by more than one disability.

As with all other outcomes, rates of disabilities increase with lowering gestational age at birth and are highest for newborns born at current limits of viability around 22 to 23 weeks of gestational age. Let's look at a few larger datasets published in the literature.

Frederik Serenius, with his colleagues, published neurodevelopmental outcomes collected from over 700 babies born in Sweden.[7] The data covers newborns born at fewer than 27 weeks between 2004 and 2007. The researchers compared important outcomes between the groups of babies born before 27 weeks and those between 37 and 41 weeks. They found that, in the group of premature babies, 64% had no intellectual disability, 61% had no language disability, and 56% had no motor disability. These values for full-term babies were 92%, 89%, and 87%, respectively. An additional finding was that 7% of premature babies were diagnosed with cerebral palsy versus only 0.1% among mature babies. Please note that for calculation purposes,

---

[7] Neurodevelopmental Outcome in Extremely Preterm Infants at 2.5 Years After Active Perinatal Care in Sweden. Fredrik Serenius et al. JAMA 2013 https://jamanetwork.com/journals/jama/fullarticle/1682943

as a denominator, researchers used the total number of survivors, not the number of births.

The French study I mentioned above in relation to survival rates also looked at outcomes.[2] The researchers analyzed data in three groups of babies: 24 to 26 weeks, 27 to 31 weeks, and 32 to 34 weeks. Rates of cerebral palsy were 6.9%, 4.3%, and 1%; rates of deafness 1.4%, 0.6%, and 0.5%; rates of blindness 0.7%, 0.3%, and 0.2% consecutively.

Let's look again at Rysavy's report,[1] which allows us to analyze adverse neurodevelopmental outcomes for each early week at birth. I want to focus our attention on severe impairment. The authors defined it as a score, which is two standard deviations below the mean on tests showing one's motor and intellectual abilities. Severe cerebral palsy, bilateral blindness, and severe hearing impairment also qualified as severe impairment in this study. For newborns who received treatment, only 15.4% at 22 weeks and 25% at 23 weeks survived without severe impairment. For babies born at 24, 25, and 26 weeks, corresponding survival rates without severe impairment were 46.1%, 61.4%, and 75.7%, respectively.

All three studies that I have used in this chapter are available freely on the internet. I have provided their links in their respective footnotes. If you have the patience for numbers and statistics, I strongly encourage you to look at them. They are rich in data and provide a granular analysis of all the results depending on varying circumstances.

Other outcomes

Following discharge from a NICU, premature babies continue to be at risk of having more health problems than their healthy term peers. Former premature babies tend to require more frequent pediatric appointments and hospital admissions because of their chronic health problems. One North-American study reported that 2% of newborns born with a birth weight of fewer than 1,000 g (2.2 lb) had died by 22 months of age following NICU discharge.

Not surprisingly, former premature babies need to see their doctors more frequently, and they are also more likely to be admitted to hospital. English scientists reported that the risk of requiring three or more hospitalizations by the age of five years for children born before 32 weeks is 13.6% versus 2.8% for full-term babies. Common reasons for rehospitalizations are respiratory syncytial virus infections, asthma, gastrointestinal problems, and issues related to chronic lung disease.

Some epidemiological studies also report that former premature babies are more likely to have problems in their adulthood related to chronic kidney diseases, high blood pressure, and decreased fertility.

Developmental evaluations

In the USA, most premature babies born before 30 weeks are referred at discharge for developmental follow-up. Skilled professionals such as developmental pediatricians, occupational therapists, and physical therapists will be seeing your baby at regular intervals to assess their motor and intellectual development. If the professionals detect any deviations from the norm and if previously not done, your baby will be referred to an early intervention program. This program aims to provide services such as occupational, physical, and speech therapy to optimize your child's development. Often, babies born before 28 weeks with IVH, BPD, severe ROP, or deafness are referred to the early intervention programs at discharge time.

In summary, I want to emphasize that your baby is a unique human being and predictions based only on past statistical data may be wrong. Your baby may have a particular set of individual circumstances that will make any prognosis that is solely based on statistics false. If you want to know the actual long-term prognosis for your baby, you need to get involved in sincere discussions with your neonatologist. I hope that my chapter on outcomes and the review of the three articles I have listed will prepare you better for such a discussion.

CHAPTER 22

Special situations— genetic syndromes and congenital anomalies

G enetic disorders and congenital anomalies affect both full-term and preterm newborns. We estimate that about 3% of all infants suffer from a genetic condition or congenital syndrome that may impair their mental or physical health. If we included in our estimates even minor malformation, up to 8% of children would be counted. It is only logical that the frequency of these conditions is likely to be slightly higher among premature babies because some will lead to early labor.

Genetics and embryology are complicated disciplines. In this chapter, I want to give you only basic information about how we approach genetic and congenital conditions. I will provide you with a few definitions and explain the diagnostic process.

Definitions

All diseases that we acquired while being created from the mother's egg and the father's sperm or during pregnancy are called "**congenital conditions.**" They include genetic conditions, malformations due to environmental or unknown random influences, and congenital infections. Congenital diseases, by definition, are always present at birth but, due to various factors, they might be recognized only many years later. Environmental factors that can lead to congenital defects include drugs, chemical exposures, and physical agents such as radiation and thermal exposures.

If an exposure to a physical or chemical factor can damage a growing embryo and fetus, we call this agent a "**teratogen.**"

"**Genetic code**" or "**genes**" can be compared to the operating system on our computer. Each cell in our body has a full set of information about us. It is written using chemical compounds (DNA) and consists of thousands of genes. When an egg gets fertilized during conception, the mother and the father pass genetic code to their offspring. However, during that process, some faulty genes or chromosomes (chromosomes = bigger chunks of genetic code) may be given to a baby, or new defective genetic information may be created.

A condition that is due to an abnormal genetic code in our body is called a "**genetic disorder**" or "**genetic syndrome.**" If a pathology found in a person is characterized by criteria that need to occur in each affected individual, we use the terms "disorder" or "disease." If a condition has a very different presentation in various people, we may prefer to use the term "**syndrome.**" For example, some people with Down syndrome will have abnormal heart anatomy and others will not. Syndromes may have a long list of possible abnormal findings. However, each affected person will manifest only some of them, and there will be considerable variability in the severity of symptoms.

A "**malformation**" is a general term used to describe abnormal anatomy or structural defects in external appearance or internal organs. One extra finger, missing fingers or hand, or a deformed ear are examples of malformations.

Diagnostic approach to congenital conditions

The approach to congenital diseases starts during the first pre-natal visit and continues throughout the whole pregnancy. First, an obstetrician gathers the history of genetic conditions in the family and any harmful environmental exposures in the mother and father of the baby. Then, some screening blood tests are done to assess the fetus's risk for a few genetic abnormalities. Finally, while doing ultrasounds during the second or third trimester, obstetricians look for structural defects in the fetus.

Despite our best efforts, many times, prenatal tests do not reveal any abnormalities, but the baby presents after birth with certain defects suggestive of congenital etiology. Whenever a newborn has more than one structural defect, we should explore genetic or teratogenic etiology. For example, if a baby has a single congenital defect in the heart called ventricular septal defect (VSD), we can attribute this to chance. However, if the same baby has VSD, a single kidney (humans typically have two kidneys), and a malformed ear, we need to consider genetic etiology.

When we have a baby who requires work-up for genetic and congenital disorders, we call on genetics specialists. After getting a comprehensive family history and examining the baby, they will order radiologic imaging studies and various blood tests. Imaging studies are done to confirm or rule out structural abnormalities in the heart, gut, kidneys, bones, or brain.

There is a multitude of genetic blood tests that we can utilize. All have a specific purpose, and a different cost and difficulty level. Some may need to be sent out to a specialized genetics lab and take a month to get results back.

After a full work-up has been completed, a genetics specialist will meet with the parents to provide results. They will explain the findings, whether they were able to identify any specific genetic defects, and what might be the prognosis for the baby. Despite our best efforts, we can only confirm a genetic etiology in 40% to 60% of babies with congenital abnormalities. It is that way because there are thousands of genes in our body, and some genetic conditions have not been discovered yet. Furthermore, some congenital malformations are due to harmful environmental exposures that can mimic genetic defects.

Treatment of congenital conditions

A lot of scientists are working on gene therapies, so in the future we might have some tools to cure genetic disorders. Currently, treatment of congenital conditions focuses on restoring optimal function of affected organs and, in many cases, will not be curative.

Curing or reversing genetic defects or environmental teratogenic effects is not possible yet. We can only address some congenital infections using antibiotics.

If a baby has abnormal anatomy of the heart or kidney, or malformed bones, surgery may be able to restore or at least improve the function of the affected organs. If a genetic condition affects the baby's intellectual capacity, special education will be required.

Questions to ask physicians if your baby is suspected of having a congenital condition

1. What makes you think that my baby has a congenital condition?
2. What are all the abnormal findings on physical examination?
3. What are all the abnormal findings on imaging studies (radiologic tests)?
4. What are all the abnormal lab tests in my baby?
5. What specialists are involved in the care of my baby, and what do they say?
6. Can I talk to the sub-specialists involved about my baby?
7. Are you doing any additional tests to diagnose my baby further?
8. Do we have a detailed prognosis related to the congenital condition that you are suspecting in my baby?
9. How are you planning to mitigate the effects of the congenital condition my baby has?

CHAPTER 23

Discharge home– when and how to prepare for it?

When can a premature baby go home from a neonatal intensive care unit?

"When can my baby go home?" is one of the most frequently asked questions when I talk to parents after admission of their baby to the neonatal intensive care unit (NICU). In this chapter, I will discuss in detail when you can expect your baby to go home without giving you an exact date for the discharge.

What are the criteria that need to be met before a premature baby can go home?

Given the number and complexity of problems that a premature baby has to deal with after birth, each baby has its unique situation and predicting a discharge date is very difficult, if not impossible. In general, most premature babies go home before their due dates. If a baby was born very early (fewer than 28 weeks of gestational age) and developed one or more complications, such a baby has a higher chance of needing hospitalization beyond its due date.

Below I list the most important criteria that neonatologists will consider before deciding whether a premature baby is ready to go home with their parents and family.

1. Ability to maintain normal body temperature in an open crib. Many premature babies after birth have problems regulating their body temperature. This occurs due to lack of energy sources, an immature brain, and the fact that room temperature is much lower than the maternal body temperature to which they were exposed in utero. We address this problem by placing babies in isolettes or incubators (an isolette is a fancy computerized plastic box in which we can regulate environmental temperature and humidity so that the baby is comfortable and will be able to maintain appropriate body temperature). All babies who are candidates to go home need to have a healthy body temperature in an open crib without too many layers of clothes or blankets for at least 48 hours before discharge.

2. The baby should have a regular breathing pattern (no clinically significant apneas: that is, short pauses in breathing). Premature babies are known to have apneas (see Chapter 9). Sometimes we treat apnea with a medication called "caffeine," and sometimes we watch it to make sure that it does not get worse. Regardless of the apnea's cause, we do not want to discharge a baby with significant apnea: therefore, that problem needs to be resolved. If the baby has been treated with caffeine, most clinicians will delay discharge home for 5 to 7 days after the medication was stopped.

3. No more significant bradycardias. The standard heart rate of a newborn is usually between 120 and 160 beats per minute. Some premature babies may have periods when their heart rate slows down to 80 per minute or lower. Such a clinical condition is called "bradycardia." Persistent or recurrent periods of bradycardia are not safe, and we would want a premature baby to outgrow that problem before discharge home.

4. A premature baby needs to be consistently gaining weight on the current nutritional schedule.

5. Stable oxygen requirement if a baby is on additional oxygen for breathing. If the baby developed broncho-pulmonary dysplasia (see Chapter 11), resulting in the prolonged need for supplementary oxygen, we some-times send such a baby home on oxygen provided that the amount of oxygen needed is not very high and does not fluctuate a lot during the day and night.

6. If your baby is receiving gavage nasogastric, orogastric or gastronomy tube feedings, you need to be comfortable with providing these feedings at home. Unfortunately, some babies, particularly those who were extremely premature or born as micro-preemies, have a hard time to learn how to eat by mouth using a bottle. In these sit-uations, we can send babies home provided that parents and all caretakers have learned how to give feedings using various tubes and are comfortable with such solutions.

7. If a baby requires special equipment (e.g. oxygen tanks, monitors, tubes, dressings) at home, all that needs to be ordered and delivered to the parents' house, and the par-ents need to learn how to use it.

8. If a baby needs any medications after discharge, the pre-scriptions should have been written and filled, and the parents taught how to administer them to their baby.

9. All acute and chronic problems that a baby has been suf-fering from should have been resolved or stabilized, so

that there is no more need for continuous or frequent monitoring or laboratory testing.

10. Sub-specialty doctors should clear a baby for discharge and indicate whether they need to see the baby in outpatient clinics for follow-ups.
11. Parents have to feel that they are ready to take their baby home. That involves a lot of learning. Parents should be able to feed the baby without problems. They need to demonstrate that they know how to use all the necessary equipment and how to give medications to their baby.

As you can see, the decision to send a premature baby home from a NICU is very complicated and must be individualized. Each newborn baby has a different set of medical problems, and each family has a distinct ability to learn the tasks needed to take care of the baby. Healthcare providers need to be able to adjust their decisions to those factors.

Is there a specific weight that a baby needs to achieve before going home from a neonatal intensive care unit?

It may be surprising to you, but there is no specific weight criterion for a baby to go home from a NICU. But they must be mature enough, and all essential vital organs such as the lungs, heart, digestive system, and central nervous system must be functioning so that it is safe for the baby to be at home with their family. The best indicators of such maturity are signs that the baby is:

- feeding without difficulties;
- gaining weight;
- breathing regularly;
- having a regular heart rate; and
- able to maintain their normal body temperature in an open crib.

What to do if I am scared to take my baby home?

It is common for parents to want their baby home as soon as possible but then, when that day is around the corner, to feel scared and have doubts. Parents always question themselves if they will be able to do everything right. The best solution is to visit your baby very often during their NICU stay. Try to learn as much as you can from NICU nurses. Specifically, learn how to:

- hold your baby correctly;
- change their diaper;
- do their bath;
- give them their medications; and
- feed them:

Feeding a premature baby differs from feeding a full-term baby and may take a long time to learn. Share your doubts with your baby's nurses and doctors so they can reassure you and support you as much as you need. Finally, doctors can arrange for a home healthcare nurse to visit you at home. They will check on your baby and address any questions and problems you may have after taking your baby home.

How to prepare for a premature baby getting discharged home from the neonatal intensive care unit?

In this section, I will advise what you should consider doing before your baby's discharge.

Check if your insurance covers your baby

If you have private health insurance from your employer, you probably know that you can renew it or make changes only once a year during the enrollment period, usually in November. However, if you have a baby, you can add your baby to your insurance after birth (there may be a time window that you need to be aware of). If you have a choice between two different insurance companies (mother's and father's), review carefully which policy will be better for your baby from a financial point of view, and which one will give better access to any doctors that your baby will need to see after discharge home.

If your family does not have private health insurance, contact the hospital case manager as soon as possible to discuss whether Medicaid can cover your baby. If you are eligible, you should sign up for Medicaid as quickly as possible.

Finish any pending home projects

Commonly, parents plan to remodel their house or room for the baby. Unfortunately, any remodeling is associated with dirt, dust, and the smell of various chemicals—not an ideal environment for a newborn baby and even less so for a premature baby. If you have not done all the necessary home improvement projects yet and your baby will be coming home in 2 weeks, in my opinion, it is better to defer those projects until your child is over 1 or 2 years old. You want to allow enough time for all vapors of glues, chemicals, and paints to be removed from the house. It always takes more time than you think.

Make sure you have all supplies

Make a list of all the items you need to buy for your baby. The absolute essentials are:

- a crib;
- a mattress;
- blankets;
- sheets;
- clothes;
- appropriately sized diapers;
- skin moisturizer;
- cream for diaper rash;
- formula or breast milk fortifier, if applicable;
- a breast pump, if applicable;

- a breast milk warmer, if desired;
- a changing table or space; and
- a set-up for giving a bath.

Choose a pediatrician.

You need to find a pediatrician. Check that you are comfortable with their location. Find out how much access you will have to the doctor after hours. Ask also if they feel comfortable taking care of former premature babies. Finally, confirm that your pediatrician is within a network covered by your health insurance, so that you are not exposed to additional copayments and deductibles.

Find out about any additional medical appointments needed for your baby

If your baby still has some unresolved chronic medical problems that need to be followed by sub-specialists, determine who those doctors are and where their clinics are. Is it going to be easy for you to get there? Does your health insurance plan cover them? We doctors tend to send babies for follow-up to the doctors within the university network where we work and know everybody. This does not mean that you cannot take your baby somewhere else for future outpatient appointments if you want to.

Sometimes you may have better specialists closer to your house. If you want to consider different options for post-discharge appointments, just discuss these with the healthcare team taking care of your baby in the NICU.

Learn all the skills needed to take care of your baby

While your baby is in the NICU, visit them as much as you can. Each time, try to participate in anything that their nurse allows you to do. Learn how to feed and burp your baby, change their diapers, take their temperature, or give them a bath. Learn how to draw medications and how to give them to your baby.

Whenever you are in the NICU, observe your baby—paying attention to their breathing patterns and skin color. Try to recognize signs of trouble, if any (turning blue, pause in breathing, choking, etc.). All these skills will be invaluable once you are on your own with the baby at home. Even if you had previously taken care of full-term babies, be aware that taking care of a premature baby is very different.

Fill all the prescriptions

If your premature baby is sent home on medications, make sure that you have already filled prescriptions, and you know how to draw them and administer them. It is also a good idea to know what these medications are for, and to be familiar with their potential side effects. If you have other children at home, make sure that you have a safe place to store the medications to prevent any accidental ingestion and poisoning.

Learn how to use all medical equipment

If your baby is sent home on oxygen, monitors, or nasogastric or gastronomy tube feedings, make sure that you are very comfortable operating them. Learn well how to use them, how to troubleshoot, and whom to call in the case of malfunctioning equipment and the urgent need to solve the problem.

Consider your financial and job situation

Having a baby is a joy, but it is also associated with additional expenses for the family budget. Having a premature baby adds to your costs even more. Families have to consider all the implications of having one parent stay at home to take care of their child. Making such decisions will require considering what it would cost them to lose one income and how much it would cost to hire help. If the mother is a single parent, these choices are even more difficult. If you or your family are going through financial hardships, talk to the hospital social worker to explore any assistance programs you might be eligible for.

Who will be taking care of your baby at home?

Even if the mother or father plans to stay at home to look after their baby, sometimes they will need a break. There will be times when you will want to have somebody else to be familiar with your child. You will need to feel safe to leave the baby in their care while you take needed rest or attend to some matters for which you have to leave the house.

Learn how to resuscitate a newborn or infant in case of an emergency

It is recommended that you and all caretakers learn how to resuscitate a baby and infant. In the rare case of emergency, when your baby turns blue or starts choking, you should know what to do and how to help them. If not offered to you by the NICU, call around and ask where you can learn these essential skills. You can probably find a cardiorespiratory resuscitation (CPR) course by calling your local fire station or police station. You can also search for CPR courses on the American Heart Association website (https://www.heart.org). To find CPR classes, click on the link; then, under the CPR tab, click on "find training center" and enter your address or zip code.

Quit smoking cigarettes

If you or somebody else in the house is a smoker, now is the time to quit. Sign up for programs that can help you with that. Cigarette smoke and other pollutants may trigger breathing problems and possibly sudden infant death syndrome in former premature babies.

Ask about vaccinations

Your baby will be getting some vaccinations during their first year of life. However, due to prematurity, your little one will be more sensitive to acquiring or becoming very sick from exposure to various bacteria and viruses. Ask your neonatologist which vaccinations are recommended for you, your family, and other caretakers. Usually, we recommend that adults and children around your baby are current with 'flu shots, and pertussis (whooping cough), chickenpox, and MMR vaccinations.

Relax and take a deep breath!

Finally, you need to relax a little bit and try not to be scared. It is a very joyful moment when your baby is finally coming home. If in doubt, ask your doctors, nurses, or therapists for help.

CHAPTER 24

Final remarks

I f you have got to this chapter, it probably means that you have read the whole book, or your baby is getting discharged home. Thank you, and congratulations. You have just passed the first milestone on a very long journey. Bringing up a child is always a great responsibility but taking care of a former premature baby is even more challenging.

I want to share a few final thoughts with you. I know you are worried about the future. Remember that no matter what your doctors told you and what statistics are predicting for your baby, these are just numbers and your baby is a unique human being. Reality is often very different from our or doctors' expectations. You have a lot to offer to your child. Your ability to take care and developmentally stimulate your baby will have an enormous impact on their future outcomes.

Make sure that you involve other people who can help: pediatricians, nurses, developmental specialists, occupational therapists (OTs), physical therapists (PTs), and, most importantly, family members. I believe that knowledge gives you power. Read books on child development and how to stimulate it. Learn from OTs, PTs, and other specialists in development. Because you and your family members will be spending the most time with your child, you will have the most significant impact on their development.

If you are a first-time mother or father, I encourage you to talk to your parents and get their perspective on how to bring up a child. Read books (there are plenty) about your child's first year. All this will be invaluable to you.

Before we say final goodbyes, I want to give you some safety guidelines to prevent adverse outcomes at home. The list is not all-inclusive, but it is a good start. You should always think about safety first: is there anything that could threaten your baby or other children's well-being? I encourage you to read through the list and talk to your trusted neonatologist and pediatrician. Make sure that they agree with it and allow them to add different items specific to your situation.

Safety guidelines for newborn babies going home:

1. When leaving your baby in their crib, always place them on their back. Infants should sleep only on their back (unless there are medical reasons for different sleeping positions)! Babies who sleep on their back are less likely to have sudden infant death syndrome (SIDS).
2. Remove soft and loose bedding and stuffed toys from your baby's sleep area. Your baby does not need a pillow. Always leave your baby's face uncovered.
3. Do not let your baby get too warm while sleeping.
4. Do not let your baby sleep in bed with you or with anyone else.
5. While feeding, always hold your baby—do not prop up the bottle.
6. Burp your baby often, both during and after feeding.
7. Avoid shaking your baby; do not change suddenly their position or press their stomach after feeding.
8. Make sure that the bathwater temperature is not too warm.
9. Never leave your baby alone during their bath.
10. During a bath, always support your baby's head and shoulders.

11. Never leave your baby alone on unsecured surfaces such as tables. Even if you think babies cannot roll over, they do!
12. Use an appropriate car seat for your baby's size and your car.
13. Do not smoke in the house and, even better, quit smoking.
14. If you leave your baby sleeping alone in another room, make sure they are safe from other small children and home pets.
15. If your baby did not have any infections and you did not read <u>Chapter 18</u>, please read the section on respiratory syncytial virus (RSV). RSV can affect former premature babies and I would like you to know about this virus

I want to thank you again for reading my book. I am hoping that it was useful. I have put a lot of effort into preparing it, and I would like to improve future editions. Please share your suggestions with me. If you wish that I covered some topics with more detail or if you think certain parts are too complicated, please let me know. You can send me your comments directly to: info@neopededu.com or reach me on my Facebook page—NeoPedEdu.

Finally, if you don't mind, share some positive comments on the portal where you purchased the book. I will be very grateful for that. This book addresses a tiny market (niche market), and it isn't easy to find by those who need it. Often book portals do not show a book in search results unless it has plenty of reviews or people are looking for the specific title.

Thank you,
W.M. WIsniewski.

About the author

Wlodzimierz M. Wisniewski MD, MHPE

Dr Wlodzimierz M Wisniewski was born in Poland. He graduated from Poznan Medical School in Poland in 1991 and then completed four years of pediatric and neonatal training in Kalisz Children's Hospital (Poland). During that time, he obtained Polish Board Certification in Pediatrics.

In 1995, he came to the USA, where he trained and practiced pediatrics and neonatology. He completed residency training in pediatrics in 1998 and a fellowship in neonatal–perinatal medicine in 2001 at the University of Illinois at Chicago (UIC). Dr Wisniewski holds the American Board of Pediatrics' certifications in both specialties. During his medical training at the UIC, he also completed a Master's degree in health professionals' education (MHPE).

After his training, from 2001 onwards, Dr Wisniewski worked in several university and community hospitals in Illinois and North Carolina as a neonatologist, medical director, and quality improvement leader. Over the past five years, Dr Wisniewski has been professionally associated with Northwestern University Health System and Lurie Children's Hospital in Chicago, Illinois.

www.ingramcontent.com/pod-product-compliance
Lightning Source LLC
Chambersburg PA
CBHW070804280326
41934CB00012B/3057